Responsive Dementia Care

Fewer Behaviors
Fewer Drugs

Helen Whitworth, MS, BSN

James A. Whitworth, LBDA co-founder

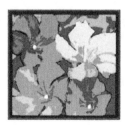

Oleander Books

Educate, Engage
Empower

Other books by the Whitworths

A Caregiver's Guide to Lewy Body Dementia (2010). An award-winning overview of Lewy body dementia and how to deal with it.... *"most helpful...field guide for caring for someone with Lewy Body!"* One of over 130 five-star Amazon.com reviews.

Riding a Rollercoaster with Lewy Body Dementia (2009). A textbook for staff. ...*"easy to understand but thorough. I learned so much."* A registered nurse.

Managing Cognitive Issues in Parkinson's and Lewy Body Dementia (2015). ...*"first book I read when we began to suspect more than PD. ...calming for a new caregiver."* Amazon.com review.

Books by Helen Buell Whitworth

On the Road with the Whitworths: A Thrifty Couple's Tribulations and Triumphs (2015). Humorous experiences while RVing in their "new" motor home. *"I loved it. It was hilarious."* Reader's review.

Betsy (2nd ed., 2014, 1st ed., 2006) A novel based on Helen's family history. *"I couldn't put it down."* Reader's review.

The Northwest McCutchens: Generation One. (2017) Facts presented in novel fashion. *"I love your books."* Family member reader's review.

The Northwest McCutchens: The Exodus. (2018) Just out. The continued story of James and Mary McCutchen.

All books are available on Amazon or LBDtools.com.

Contents

INTRODUCTION TO RESPONSIVE CARE 1

SECTION ONE: DOING THE RESEARCH.......................................5

   1. DEMENTIA-RELATED BEHAVIORS 7

   2. DRUGS AND DRUG SENSITIVITY.................................... 23

   3. THE SENSES.. 35

   4. THINKING SKILLS 43

   5. PERCEPTUAL DYSFUNCTIONS 59

   6. EMOTIONS 65

   7. IMPULSES AND DISINHIBITION.................... 71

   8. STRESS 75

   9. MOOD DISORDERS.................................... 87

SECTION TWO: PUTTING THE CARE PARTNER FIRST.............97

   10. BASIC NEEDS 99

   11. CAREGIVING IS NOT A ONE-PERSON JOB 109

   12. BECOME AN IMPROV ACTOR 117

   13. BEING FLEXIBLE 129

   14. BEING POSITIVE 137

   15. RESPITE.. 147

SECTION THREE: PROVIDING THE CARE 151

   16. BEING A TEAM.................................... 153

   17. BEING PERSON-CENTERED 161

   18. BEING ACCEPTING 167

   19. WORKING WITH PRESENT ABILITIES 173

   20. BEING EMPATHETIC.................................... 179

   21. BEING ENGAGING.................................... 185

   22. KEEPING TRACK 199

SECTION FOUR: ALTERNATIVE OPTIONS 203

23. REHABILITATIVE THERAPIES 205

24. PREVENTIVE MEASURES 211

25. HEALTHY LIVING PRACTICES 219

26. RELAXATION EXERCISES 227

27. USING THE SENSE PATHWAYS.............................. 231

28. ENHANCING ACTIVITIES 245

29. SPORTS, GAMES, HOBBIES, SPECIAL INTERESTS 255

SUMMING IT UP... 259

RESOURCES 261

GLOSSARY.. 269

REFERENCES... 287

About the Cover

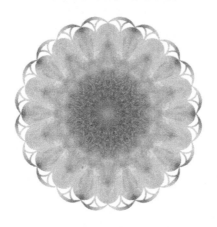

We chose this beautiful mandala for our cover because it fits with our work in several ways. Like snowflakes and people living with dementia, each mandala is unique. Like a person living with dementia, a mandala's convoluted lines can be confusing. On the other hand, tracing the lines of a mandala can be calming. I found this one called "alien brain" during a search for brain images which we had considered. Well, that title fits too--as dementia advances it does seem alien at times!

Dedication

We dedicate this book to the many care partners who willingly put their lives on hold to care for loved ones living with dementia. We write for those who find themselves in a not-so-merry-go-round of interactions with a once-rational person where old and tried responses trigger new and confusing dementia-related behaviors. And we speak for those who have had negative experiences with behavior management drugs and need other options.

Acknowledgments

We have so many people to thank for the information in this book. Way back in 2006, we watched Dr. Tanis Ferman's presentation on behavioral challenges at the Many Faces of Lewy Body Dementia conference. That was the start. Since then, we've discovered the wonderful work of Teepa Snow and her Positive Approach. We also need to thank all of those who have shown how effective improv acting can be with dementia. Then, there are the many alternative therapists like our friend, Regina Hucks, who taught us about other non-drug options for care. Of course, we couldn't have done this book without all the care partners who shared their experiences with us--and our readers. Last but far from least, we thank the people who helped to make this book readable: Leanne Buell, Rosemary Dawson, Pat Snyder, Connie Hanna, and many other reviewers. To all who helped to make this book what it is, your work has been greatly appreciated

About the Authors

James and Helen Whitworth have been teaching and writing about Lewy body dementia for over a decade. James is a retired electrical engineer. When his first wife, Annie, had Lewy body dementia (LBD) in the late 1990's, he had no idea of how to deal with the behavioral symptoms of her disorder. Sadly, neither did her doctors who treated her symptoms with drugs that often caused more problems than they fixed.

James experienced many of the trials that care partners report regularly in online and local LBD support groups. After Annie passed, James joined with four other caregivers to start the Lewy Body Dementia Association (lbda.org) in 2003 and was their first board president. By the time his term on the board ended, he had met Helen.

Helen has worked in care facilities and been a family caregiver as well. With degrees in both nursing and psychology, she uses her interest in science to learn how the body functions and her interest in psychology to gain insights into personal interactions.

After she and James were married in 2005, they started working together on his mission. Since then, they've written four books and taught about Lewy body disorders and dementia in general to support groups, college classes, workshops, care facilities, medical conventions and more.

Responsive Dementia Care

Fewer Behaviors

Fewer Drugs

Introduction to Responsive Care

dementia related behaviors *(behavioral and psychological symptoms of dementia--BPSD)." Behaviors brought about by the cognitive and psychological symptoms of dementia.*

care partner: *The primary family caregiver. Called care partner to signify that caring is a team project.*

care person: *A general term for anyone providing care.*

dementia: *At least two cognitive functions so impaired that one's ability to perform activities of daily living is affected.*

LBD: Lewy body dementia, disease or disorder*: Your choice. We prefer "disease" or "disorder" because LBD impairs more than just cognition.*

Person: *The Person living with dementia, the care partner's "loved one," the nurse's "patient," the care staff's "resident," the researcher's "subject." Or use **your Person's name**.*

responsive care. *The use of knowledge, attitude, action and self-care to predict, prevent, change or encourage a Person's behavior and maintain the care partner's effectiveness.*

alternative options: *Non-drug remedies and interventions used alone or in combination with drug therapy. Includes communication skills, stress management, and a variety of rehabilitative, preventive, and enhancing therapies.*

takeaways: *The summary lists of information, attitudes, actions and self-care ideas at the end of each chapter helpful for performing responsive care.*

***

Difficult behaviors usually show up eventually with all dementias. However, they are especially frustrating for anyone dealing with Lewy body disorders (LBD) because:

- Behaviors tend to show up early while memory is still intact.
- Traditional behavior management drugs are more problematical with LBD than with other dementias.

Behaviors such as delusions, combativeness, verbal accusations, and paranoia are among the most common subjects of discussion in caregiver support groups.

"I just don't know how to deal with Gerry's hallucinations. I used to be able to tell him they weren't real but now he gets mad when I try to explain. What am I doing wrong? -- Olivia

Olivia is stuck wanting "what is" to be "what was." As dementia takes its toll, a Person's reality changes. When the care partner isn't responsive to this change, there will be conflict. Sometimes the situation is more critical than just conflict, which can be painful enough.

Mason still wants to drive. I know it doesn't do any good to reason with him. I told him I was afraid to ride with him anymore and that didn't work either. I don't know what to do. -- Iris

Iris is one step closer to responsive caring. She knows what **not to do**, but she doesn't know what **to do**. She knows not to argue with Mason but she still doesn't know how to defuse the situation.

Basic caregiving skills aren't enough. Because of issues like Olivia's and Iris's, there's much more to being a dementia care partner than knowing how to do the physical caregiving.

Responsive caring speaks to this by responding to the Person's emotional needs, rather than reacting to their behaviors. The difference between reacting and responding is that reacting is an automatic, usually defensive action. Responding is a thought-out response, based on knowledge of the situation and a goal for the future.

Responsive caring is a multi-part process:

Learning about such things as:

- How dementia changes the brain, the specific type of dementia involved and the Person's unique expression of it.
- Stress and how it is connected with behaviors.
- Behavior management drugs along with their effectiveness and issues.
- Alternative options for behavior management along with their effectiveness and issues.

Attitudes such as these:

- Awareness: being alert for changes and needs, being aware of your own emotions and needs.
- Acceptance: accepting "what is" instead of what you would like it to be; accepting the Person's needs for personhood, validation, respect and belief; accepting your own vulnerabilities.
- Empathy: Seeing events from the Person's viewpoint; experiencing what they feel.
- Patience: Relaxing, slowing down.
- Calmness: Keeping the intensity down.
- Optimism, gratitude, hopefulness and positive attitudes that make the job easier and more pleasant.

Actions that:

- Support the Person's need to feel validated, respected and cared about.
- Are more likely to move the action forward with the fewest problems.

Self-care that:

- Supports the idea that the care partner is the most important dementia care tool.
- Protects and supports the care partner's ability to provide the best care they can.

Responsive caring doesn't happen overnight. You may have had to start being a care partner quickly, but it takes time to learn the information, make the changes in attitude and develop the skills. Because dementia is ever-changing, responsive care also involves being responsive to these irrevocable changes, accepting them and adapting to them while recognizing still-present abilities.

Responsive caring is not a panacea, a fix-all. Behaviors will still occur, but they will be fewer and less intense than they would be otherwise. The dementia will still progress, but life will be much more enjoyable for both the care partner and the Person.

You may notice that this book includes some repetition. The book is designed to introduce topics early on with short examples and expand on them in later chapters. This leads to repetition, especially of that information we consider important. For example, the definition for alternative options is in two chapters and the glossary. This means that you don't have to go back to check it out. And if you are an already-stressed care partner, the repetition help with remembering information.

Section One: Doing the Research

Responsive care starts with building a knowledge base. The more you know about how dementia changes your loved one, the better you will be able to provide the care they need. Care persons are usually much more interested in learning how to deal with dementia's disturbing behaviors than in learning why those behaviors occur. However, knowing the whys of a behavior adds reason and thus, helps the care person to find a solution, often intuitively.

For example, if you know that a Person is acting super dependent out of fear of abandonment, it is reasonable to help them to feel secure rather than to try to escape their incessant shadowing. If you know that their view of a situation is unchangeable, it is reasonable to flow with it rather than try to convince them to change. If you know that certain events trigger negative feelings and that negative feelings trigger negative behaviors, it is reasonable to do your best to avoid those triggering events.

And then, surprise! The time you take to learn about the whys and the effort you make to put them into practice causes care to be easier, less time consuming, more pleasant and more rewarding.

Knowledge is power. It gives you the insight needed to develop supportive responses to the Person's often confusing behaviors. It provides a basis on which to build responsive caring.

Without it, you are likely to struggle on, reacting to the Person's behaviors in the ways that become increasingly less effective as dementia advances. In the past, this is when a greater use of drugs often occurred along with their unwanted side effects.

With knowledge, you can let go of expectations that have made your efforts ineffective and even disruptive and develop attitudes that encourage a Person to feel accepted and open the way to better communication.

With knowledge, you can choose from a variety of less risky but often equally effective alternative behavior management methods, including healthy living practices, stress management tools, improv acting, empathetic communication and a variety of rehabilitative, preventive, and enhancing therapies.

With knowledge, you will take better care of yourself. You will know you are your Person's most important tool in their battle with dementia. Since you want them to have the most effective tools possible, you will view your efforts to be healthy, happy and capable as an integral part of your job.

1. Dementia-Related Behaviors

dementia-related behaviors (behaviors): *The Person's behavioral and psychological responses to perception, thought and mood disturbances.*

triggers: *Conditions that cause the Person to exhibit unwanted behaviors.*

Dementia-related behaviors are often a form of stress-related communication. They become more common as the ability to think abstractly fades. This happens early with LBD, but occurs eventually with all dementias. Behaviors can also be organic, caused by the disease itself. LBD-related apathy and depression are examples of this.

List of behaviors

Below is an introductory list of many of the behaviors most often reported in caregiver support groups or documented in the literature.[1] As you continue through this book, you will learn more about them, how they are triggered and how to deal with them.

These behavioral symptoms are listed in categories although many actually fit into more than one category. For example, most behaviors have disinhibition aspects in that they tend to be impulsive and uncontrollable. Capgras Syndrome is another example. It is a delusion brought about by damaged visual perceptions.

As you read through this list, you will likely be familiar with some and not with others. Every Person is different, with different symptoms. Where the symptoms are similar, the intensity may be different. With each symptom, look for what causes the Person's behavior and the emotions involved. That's how responsive care starts--with information.

Aggressive behavior. Can be expressed physically as combativeness or threatening behavior, or verbally as verbal aggressiveness or vocally disruptive behavior.

- *Combativeness, physical aggression and threatening behavior*: Usually expressed in reaction to perceived danger, pain or reason for anger.

Annie was always trying to hit me for no apparent reason. I didn't know how to make her stop. She wouldn't ever tell me why. In fact she didn't say much at all anymore. I'd try to avoid her and that just made her madder. -- James (Whitworth)

From James's point of view, Annie's behavior was irrational. From Annie's, it wasn't. She was trying to tell James that she was hurting and he was failing to fix it. She probably didn't know why she hurt and could no longer verbalize it if she had known.

- *Verbal aggressiveness.* An effort to communicate often made worse by frustration. Often combined with delusions of infidelity, theft or abandonment.

When Carter hears me talking to my daughter on the phone, he gets really upset and accuses me of talking to my boyfriend. --Gwen

The intensity is evidence of Carter's discomfort and fear of abandonment.

- *Resistance.* The refusal to do something the care partner considers necessary, often involving hygiene. This behavior is usually more passive-aggressive but the Person can become aggressive if the care partner persists in their demands.

My husband resists my efforts to get him to change his adult diaper even after he messes it. He's even tried to hit me when I insist. – Joan, wife of Walter

Joan isn't going to be able to convince her husband that he needs clean clothes because he probably doesn't smell or feel a problem. Resistance usually occurs when the Person feels put upon to perform acts that they consider unnecessary, uncomfortable or scary.

Delusions: Irrational beliefs that can show up very early with LBD, and later with other dementias. Delusions occur when the Person's brain attempts to make sense of sensory input and emotions without the help of abstract thinking skills. Once in place, the lack of those same skills make delusions impossible to change. This bears repeating: *The Person believes their delusions so strongly that this belief cannot be changed.* Common types include:

- *Stories,* where the Person believes they have experienced something that didn't really happen.
- *Accusations,* often of infidelity, abandonment or theft.
- *Misidentification,* where the Person believes that a familiar person or place has been replaced by an impostor. Capgras Syndrome (people) and reduplicative par-amnesia (places) are both signature Lewy body symptoms.
- *Paranoia:* A delusional fear of something or someone.

Delusions can't be changed but sometimes the Person can be reoriented using a different sense pathway, redirection or even simply time.

Disinhibition. The loss of filters for language and behavior. Most dementias erode the ability to discriminate, resulting in impulsive and often inappropriate words and behavior, with

9

no ability to understand that it isn't functional or socially correct.

- ***Eating inedible objects, putting anything in the mouth.***

Brian is like a two-year-old! Everything goes into his mouth. I have to watch him like a hawk. -- Molly

This type of disinhibition is a form of comforting and reassuring oral stimulation, normal in childhood and again in dementia, as the thinking abilities fade.

- ***Inappropriate dressing/undressing:*** Wearing the same clothes day after day; taking off clothes in public.

My father wants to wear the same shirt every day, even when they are dirty. And then he went for a walk and I found him walking around nude. "It's hot," he told me. – Ariel, daughter of Ralph

With life changing uncontrollably, wearing a well-known shirt adds security. With no impulse control or ability to identify norms, the Person will do what they feel is most comfortable or most familiar.

- ***Vocally disruptive behavior.*** Using inappropriate language in inappropriate places, often at a high volume.

My mother was always so prim and proper. We were just sitting in a booth in a restaurant and I couldn't believe the words that came out of her mouth. She started cussing-- loudly. This isn't the first time. I'm almost afraid to take her out in public anymore. -- Arlene, daughter of Clara

Without filters, Arlene's mother says the first thing that comes to mind. Persons are usually anxious in public situations and so she is trying to express that. Since forbidden words are stored in a part of the brain that stays functional longer than other language centers do, that's what comes out.

- *Inappropriate sexual behavior, hyper-sexuality:* Making sexual advances in public, being over-demanding with one's sexual partner.

We were visiting with a couple we've known for a long time and Brian suddenly reached out, patted the woman's breast and told her, "Nice boobs." I was mortified. -- Molly

As feelings become more important and impulse control disappears, a Person may simply act out their thoughts. Hyper-sexuality is the doing of what feels good sexually without other considerations.

- *Inappropriate urination/defecation.* Incontinence occurs with any dementia eventually but LBD damaged sphincter control can cause it to happen early on. However, even when incontinence is not an issue, a Person may not wait or want to use the toilet, or may not clean up properly.

Joe isn't really incontinent, but he will pee anywhere, in a flower pot, against the wall, whatever. He usually does use the toilet for pooping, but sometimes, he has an accident. Then he makes it worse by smearing feces all over the wall. -- Alice

With poor sphincter control, Joe has to urinate soon after he gets the urge; with little inhibition, he does so no matter where he is. The smearing was likely an effort to clean up after himself.

Perceptual disturbances

Most of these symptoms occur when the visual cortex is damaged.

- *Capgras Syndrome and reduplicative par-amnesia.* (See delusions.)

- *Disorientation due to poor depth perception.* Poor depth perception is a common LBD symptom that throws off a Person's ability to judge distances.

Dad has trouble finding his coffee cup. Then when he finally gets it in his hand, he often spills it because for some reason, he can't seem to get it up to his mouth. – Neal, Dan's son.

Dan lacks hand-eye coordination, a type of depth perception that helps him judge the distance between his hand and something else he sees. He may also have poor spatial perception which causes him to bump into tables or stumble when going from one type of flooring to another, such as from carpeting to vinyl flooring.

- *Hallucinations, visual:* Seeing something that isn't really there. Often one of the first Lewy-body-related symptoms, but common later on in other dementias as well.

I could tell when Lilburn was hallucinating by watching his eyes. Sometimes he would smile or laugh and I would ask him what he was looking at. Often, he saw small children playing under the table. This didn't disturb him, but sometimes he was worried about them getting hurt. -- Rosemary

Dementia-related hallucinations are usually benign and can be more disturbing to the care partner than to the Person experiencing them.

Sometimes, Lilburn would become very agitated when he saw home invaders carrying weapons. His adrenalin increased as he went into fight mode. "Ro, get down now so that they don't see you!" -- Rosemary

Hallucinations can sometimes be very scary. This most often occurs when combined with post traumatic stress disorder or after watching an exciting or disturbing TV program.

- *Hallucinations, other than visual.* These can be any other sense such as hearing, taste or tactile. Instead of the visual cortex, the area of the brain related to that particular sense is affected. Non-visual hallucinations are not specific LBD symptoms although they can occur.

- *Illusions.* Illusions differ from hallucinations in that there is actually something there to see, but it is perceived as something else.

Our living room carpet is flowered. Ken sees the flowers as small animals. I'd consider getting rid of the carpet but they seem to be more company for him than a bother. -- Kathy

Like hallucinations, illusions are seldom worrisome. Illusions are not considered unique LBD symptoms but they still occur commonly.

- *Mirroring:* Mirroring is actually something everyone does. We learn by mirroring behaviors and we all pick up each other's emotions.

Yesterday, I got upset about how my cake turned out. Leon picked that up and started yelling at me. – Carla

Mirroring, especially of emotions, becomes a disruption when it isn't processed properly. Randy picked up Trudy's anger, but then he owned it instead of recognizing it as neither his nor directed towards him.

Memory Loss Disturbances

Behaviors related to memory loss are often more common with Alzheimer's or mixed dementias than with LBD alone.

- *Poor personal hygiene and grooming:* Forgetting, losing interest or resisting in basic activities such as bathing, hair care and tooth brushing. Common with all dementias.

The cause for this can be varied, but includes a loss of memory about these necessary actions and little-to-no understanding of their value and social importance.

Brian resists taking a shower until he gets so grungy and actually smelly that I insist. Then he complains that it's too soon, that he says he "showered already today." -- Molly

With little concept of time, it can feel as though last week's shower was only an hour ago. Fading smell and sight can make it difficult to see a problem. Being unclothed in a cold bathroom can be scary and uncomfortable.

- *Repeating questions, often several times.* Can also repeat statements.

Roger will ask me a question and I'll answer him. Then a few minutes later, he asks the same question again. He'll tell me something over and over too. -- Jackie

Fred likely doesn't remember the previous conversation so he still feels in need of a response.

- *Task-related memory loss.* The inability to remember how to do once easy tasks. This is an executive skills-related loss, and very common for Persons living with LBD.

Annie was a great cook, but she started giving me "burnt offerings" for supper. -- James

Such losses can be quite frustrating, leading to other behaviors, or as in Annie's case, seriously dangerous. Annie had forgotten how to use the stove. She could have burned the house down instead of just the food!

- *Wandering.* Leaving the safety of known areas and getting lost. Isn't specifically a repetitive activity, but once begun, a Person will do it often.

Janie got lost driving home from the store yesterday. I finally took my car and went looking for her. She had gone off in the totally opposite direction from our home. -- Randy

Wandering can include getting lost while walking too. Because getting lost is related to memory, wandering is common with Alzheimer's where memory loss is an early symptom. However, it can show up with LBD when both types of dementia are present.

Mood Disorders

These include apathy, depression and lack of empathy. All three can present as withdrawn, uninterested, uncaring and unmotivated. They are often mistaken for each other and can appear alone or with any or all of the others.

- *Apathy.* The loss of motivation and interest in life. This is usually organic, or directly related to the disease, rather than a response to stimuli or emotions.

Fred used to be so energetic and excitable. During football season, he'd stomp and yell at the TV and the players. Now he is very low-key and shows little interest even in things like the football games that he used to love. -- Emma

Apathy often accompanies depression, especially when it is organic, but can appear alone as well.

- *Depression:* Persistent feelings of sadness, hopelessness, pessimism and a loss of interest in pleasurable activities.

Fred's depression started right after his diagnosis of LBD. -- Emma

Situational depression due to unwelcome changes in life circumstances can be fairly short-lived and can disappear as one adapts to the changes. This is often present in care partners too.

Fred and I worked through that but then the depression came back, even stronger than before. He's more apathetic now too. -- Emma

Organic depression, caused by disease-related chemical changes in the body, can be longer lasting and is often accompanied by apathy. This is especially common with LBD.

- ***Empathy deficit:*** The inability to understand or feel what another person is experiencing or feeling.

I fell down and Leon just stood there and looked at me. He didn't ask if I was all right or offer to help me up. -- Carla

Leon simply saw Carla lying on the floor. He wasn't able to experience her fear or pain. The same is true for when he might say hurtful things to her. He will not see them as hurtful to her, only to him.

Repetitive Activity

Saying or doing the same thing over and over, often compulsively. Includes such behaviors as repeating questions, hiding/hoarding food or articles, picking/tugging at things. Compulsive repetition can happen due to inability to remember, as an effort to make sense of one's fading world or as a sign of anxiety or discomfort.

- ***Agitation:*** Anxiousness expressed with restlessness, pacing, irritability and repetitive behaviors. Agitation is a part of most repetitive behaviors and a common component of other behaviors as well.

When Steve can't seem to be still, I know he's anxious. He'll pace, wring his hands or follow me around. It's usually when something unfamiliar is going on...or when he just doesn't feel good. -- Rhonda

- ***Hiding/hoarding food or articles:*** Compulsively saving items.

My mother stores bread crusts and bits of candy in her wheelchair in the nursing home and then forgets that they are there. It doesn't do any good to tell her to leave it on her plate or throw it out. She just ignores me. – Lillian, daughter of Pamela

This may be an attempt to maintain some control over all the uncontrollable losses in her life. Even if she remembered Lillian's instructions, her negative feelings of anxiety will likely be stronger than her waning need to conform to polite society.

- ***Picking or tugging at things***. Compulsively focusing on a single thing...bed clothes, hair, a sleeve, etc.

Sandy sits in her wheelchair and pulls at the threads in the afghan that covers her legs. I guess we are fortunate; another woman in her facility is continually pulling at her hair. -- Mitchell

Such repetitive behavior is usually a sign of anxiety or discomfort. When combined with other symptoms it can also be a sign that end of life is near.

- ***Shadowing.*** The attempt to keep the care partner in sight at all times.

I feel suffocated! Tony follows me everywhere. I can't turn around without bumping into him. I can't even go to the bathroom alone anymore. If I try, Tony bangs on the door until I open it. -- Angela

Like other repetitive activities, shadowing is a sign of anxiousness due to his dementia-related losses. He depends on Angela to keep him oriented and feeling safe.

Sleep Disorders

Symptoms involving sleep that result in behaviors, lack of sleep or disrupted sleep patterns and increased stress.

- *Sleep apnea:* Temporary loss of breath during sleep. Apnea due to upper respiratory obstruction is common with all dementias and the elderly in general. Apnea due to a sluggish autonomic nervous system is a common LBD symptom.

Leon tossed and turned during his sleep and I thought he was having active dreams. But they did some tests and it turned out that he was experiencing sleep apnea. The doctor prescribed a device for him to wear but he won't use it. -- Carla

Sleep apnea symptoms can be similar to active dreams, but the treatment is different. The mask used for sleep apnea can feel foreign and a Person may have difficulty understanding its value.

- *Circadian rhythm sleep disorder (CRSD).* Disruption of one's normal sleep/wake rhythm. Dementia can interfere with a Person's internal clock's ability to function properly. Because there may be no extended sleep time, the quality sleep needed for adequate rest may be missed, leading to fatigue-related stress.

Brian sleeps off and on all day and then at night, he wants to get up and wander around. I'm worn out because of always having to get up and talk him into going back to bed. Then when I finally get back in bed, I'm not sleepy anymore! -- Molly

It may also cause fatigue-related stress for the care partner when their normal sleep time is disrupted by the wide awake Person.

18

- *Sundowning.* A type of Circadian rhythm disorder where poor internal clock management brings about confusion and behaviors in late afternoon and early evening.

Mom acts perfectly normal until about four o'clock in the afternoon. Then she gets confused and stays that way for the rest of the day. I've learned to plan our outings so that she can get home before that. – Arlene, daughter of Clara

- *Excessive daytime sleeping.* A form of Circadian rhythm disorder, especially common with Parkinson's and LBD, where the Person is unable to remain awake and alert during normal waking hours. They may or may not sleep well at night.

Ellen seems to get enough sleep at night, but she sleeps during the day too. Is this all right? Should I be trying to get her to stay awake more? -- Roy

The Person with adequate nighttime sleep who still sleeps much of the day can be more worrying to the care partner than bothersome for the Person. Living with dementia is hard work; a Person may simply need that much sleep!

- *REM-sleep behavior disorder (RBD).* Also called "active dreams" for the active limb movements that occur while dreaming. This is a Lewy body disorder than can occur alone, or as a Parkinson's or LBD symptom.

Annie had active dreams for at least five years before her dementia diagnosis. She carried on involved conversations, waved her arms and once, even tried to hit me. -- James

- *Restless Leg Syndrome.* An irresistible desire to move one's legs to relieve uncomfortable sensations, usually occurring during sleep or when one's legs are at rest.

Janie often has a hard time getting to sleep. I get her into bed and all settled down and then she starts complaining about bugs crawling on her legs or sometimes she says it's "pins and needles." -- Randy

19

Unlike active dreams, restless leg syndrome is NOT a Lewy body specific symptom. It can occur alone and with most kinds of dementia. It gets worse with disturbances such as routine changes, too little sleep or too much light.

Triggers

The trigger for behaviors is usually a stressor, a stressful irritant which can be:

Physical: pain, infection or any discomfort.

External: something unpleasant seen, heard or felt.

Internal: residual negative feelings attached to a present event.

Perceptual: delusions based on failed reasoning skills.

Organic: symptoms of the disease itself, such as hallucinations or active dreams.

Combined: Most are a combination of two or more of the above. Remember Carter who overheard his wife's phone conversation with her daughter (external), experienced residual fear of abandonment and inadequacy (internal) and believed she was talking to her boyfriend (perceptual).

These stressors generate negative emotions, which in turn generate more stress. The Person acts out the stress behaviorally:

- When unable to identify the stressor, as when they are experiencing a urinary tract infection.
- When frustrated by being unable to verbally communicate and or make one's needs or wishes known.
- As a reaction to strong negative emotions such as fear or anger generated by the stressor.

Different Persons may respond with different behaviors to the same triggers. For example, in response to too much stimulation (as in too much noise) one Person may become withdrawn, while another may become irritable and even combative.

***

Responsive Care Takeaways for Dementia-Related Behaviors

- Behaviors are often a form of stress-related communication, occurring when the Person:
  - o Has difficulty expressing their needs.
  - o Feels frustration or other negative emotions build.
- Behaviors can be divided into several types although many behaviors can fit in more than one category.
  - o Aggressive behaviors: Includes combativeness, physical and verbal aggression and resistance.
  - o Delusions: Includes irrational beliefs resulting in stories, accusations, misidentification and paranoia.
  - o Disinhibition: A loss of impulse control and social filters that result in inappropriateness related to eating, dressing, words, sexual behaviors, urination and defecation.
  - o Perceptual disturbances, mostly visual, resulting in misidentification syndromes and poor depth perception, hallucinations, illusions and inaccurate mirroring.
  - o Memory loss disturbances: Poor personal care, verbal repetition, lost task-related skills and wandering.
  - o Mood disorders, including apathy, depression and lack of empathy.

- o Repetitive activities, including agitation, hoarding, compulsive picking or tugging and shadowing.
- o Sleep disorders, including apnea, Circadian rhythm sleep disorder, sundowning, excessive daytime sleeping, REM sleep behavior disorder (Active Dreams) and restless leg syndrome.
- Behaviors are usually triggered by stressful irritants that can be:
- o Physical
- o External
- o Emotional
- o Organic
- In many cases, the trigger can be a combination of two or more of these irritants.

2. Drugs and Drug Sensitivity

neurotransmitter: *A neuro (brain) chemical that transfers information from one brain cell to another.*

antipsychotics (neuroleptics): *Drugs approved for treating psychotic symptoms in psychiatric diseases such as schizophrenia and sometimes used "off label" with dementia.*

black box warning: *FDA required warning on all antipsychotic product packaging[2] that the use of antipsychotics in the elderly is linked to increased risk of serious illness and death.*

neuroleptic sensitivity: *Negative reaction to an antipsychotic drug with symptoms such as rigidity, immobility, loss of balance, difficulties with posture, sedation, and more.*

neuroleptic malignant syndrome (NMS): *Rare, possibly fatal, reaction to antipsychotic drugs, with confusion, high fever, unstable blood pressure, muscular rigidity, and autonomic dysfunction.*

anti-anxiety drugs (tranquilizers): *Drugs used to treat anxiety and agitation. Also used as muscle relaxants.*

sedatives: *Drugs used as sleeping aids and to treat anxiety.*

anticholinergic drug: *One that compromises acetylcholine. Includes muscle relaxants, anti-anxiety drugs, sedatives and antipsychotics. Most anticholinergic drugs are Lewy-sensitive.*

drug sensitivity: *The reaction to a normal dose as though it were an overdose. Varies greatly with each Person and each drug.*

dementia/Lewy-sensitive drug: *Drug that may be more sensitive with dementia in general, or specifically with LBD.*

Includes most antipsychotics, anti-anxiety drugs, sedatives and anticholinergics.

alternative options: *Non-drug remedies and interventions, including healthy living practices, stress management tools, empathetic communication and a variety of rehabilitative, preventive, and enhancing therapies. Can be used alone or in combination with drug therapy.*

Medications Glossary: *Downloadable from LBDA.org. Used along with our previous book as reference for the above drugs.*[3]

***

Drug sensitivity occurs when the body cannot metabolize or eliminate a drug in the expected amount of time. This causes the drug to become more potent and last longer, thus acting as an overdose. This can happen with most dementias, many illnesses and with age in general. It can appear fairly early in the LBD journey when Lewy bodies interfere with the brain's management of metabolization and elimination, often prior to the appearance of cognitive issues.

Lewy bodies are damaged proteins present in LBD, Parkinson's and often in mild cognitive impairment. They target certain neuro-chemicals, limiting their ability to function. Acetylcholine is a major target.

Lewy-sensitivity usually involves anticholinergic drugs, drugs that also limit acetylcholine's ability to function. The Person living with LBD gets a double hit, once from the Lewy bodies and once from the drug, greatly increasing the chances of drug sensitivity.

Most behavior management drugs are anticholinergics in addition to their intended action. Therefore, it is no wonder Persons living with LBD are often sensitive to behavior management drugs, with side effects that include heavy sedation, confusion and increased dementia symptoms. In some cases, especially with benzodiazepines such as Ativan and Xanax, there can even be an increase in the symptom the drug was supposed to treat.

In addition, drugs commonly prescribed for a variety of other uses such as muscle cramps, bladder function and mobility can also be anticholinergic, causing the same sensitivity issues as the behavior management drugs.

Antipsychotics, anti-anxiety drugs, sedatives and other mood management drugs have traditionally been used to treat dementia-related behaviors. For years, experts have recommended that, due to the above sensitivities, Persons living with LBD should be prescribed these drugs only when all else has failed. Dementia experts now advocate the use of alternative remedies first for the behaviors of all dementias and with the elderly in general.[4]

Even when behavior management drugs appear to work well, they treat the behavior, not the cause. Conversely, most alternative or non-drug options, addressed in detail in Section Four, target the cause of the behavior, so that the behavior is stopped earlier.

In support of behavior management drugs, they are usually quicker and may be more effective with less effort--when they don't cause other problems. Situations where a low dose of one of the milder drugs might be appropriate include:

- During intense or frightening behavioral episodes, such as combative or threatening behavior, to decrease the intensity enough to make alternative applications possible.

- In combination with alternative options that allow lower, safer doses and often provide better results than either used alone.

- As a short-term course given prior to a stressful event such as a trip, to decrease anticipatory stress, often worse than that of the event itself.

As with most LBD symptoms, everyone not only expresses them differently but reacts to the drugs differently.

The doctor prescribed an antipsychotic for Annie's combativeness. She quit trying to hit me, but then she had awful dreams all night long. She thrashed around so much neither of us got much rest. Her doctor prescribed a different antipsychotic and she did fine with that one. -- James

This difference makes it hard for the doctor to find the right dose--or even the right drug. It is usually a trial and error situation.

Support group discussion:

Joanne: I don't think the doctors know what they are doing. Every drug they try with Mac just makes him worse. I'm almost afraid to even give him an aspirin anymore.

Gwen: Have you tried smaller doses? That's what we did. The drug that the doctor gave Carter for hallucinations worked for a long time. And then it started making the hallucinations worse instead of better. The doctor cut his dose in half and that worked.

Doug: Nancy was doing really well. She hadn't reacted to any drugs but then she caught a cold and would you believe, she started hallucinating after I gave her an over-the-counter cold and allergy drug that we've used many times before.

As shown in the above discussion:

- Some, like Mac, are super sensitive and can tolerate very few drugs.
- Like Carter, a Person may react with unwanted symptoms but may be able to handle smaller doses.
- Even those who seem to be getting off scot-free can't expect that to continue. As it did with Nancy, the likelihood of drug sensitivity increases with the progress of the disorder.

Drug sensitivity is something that develops slowly, as more acetylcholine is compromised and as the body's waste removal system gets weaker. As such, it is hidden, showing up only when a Person reacts to some drug, often one they've taken in the past with no problem. If they are lucky, the first time will be with something like an over-the-counter cold and allergy medicine that Doug gave Nancy. These drugs are milder with a shorter half-life (the time it takes for them to become inactive).

The reaction to this milder drug is a warning to start being very careful about other drugs as well.

Usually the symptoms of drug sensitivity stop after the drug leaves the body. However, due to weakened body processes from dementia, other illness or even just age, this can take much longer than expected. With the strongest drugs the symptoms may even be permanent.

In rare cases, an extreme reaction called neuroleptic malignant syndrome (NMS) may occur. Symptoms include high fever, unstable blood pressure, muscular rigidity, autonomic dysfunction and possible death.

The following types of behavioral drugs are usually highly anticholinergic and should be avoided or used with great care and careful monitoring.

- *Antipsychotics, traditional:* First generation, used to treat psychosis such as schizophrenia. Carries a black box warning and is not FDA-approved for dementia. The only one in regular use is haloperidol (Haldol) where it is a common drug in emergency rooms and hospice services. *LBD experts recommend that these drugs **should not be given to any Person living with LBD due to the high probability of sensitivity.***

- *Benzodiazepines.* Sedative drugs with anticholinergic properties used to treat anxiety, insomnia and allergies. Should be avoided or used with extreme caution. Examples: clorazepate (Tranxene), diazepam (Valium) and alprazolam (Xanax).

- *Sleeping aids.* Sedatives with anticholinergic properties used as sleep aids. Examples: zolpidem (Ambien), eszopiclone (Lunesta) or zaleplon (Sonata).

- *Antidepressants.* First generation antidepressants are usually strong sedatives and strong anticholinergics. These drugs are seldom used anymore because there are newer, safer choices. Examples: amitriptyline (Elivil) and methyldopa (Aldomet), phenelzine (Nardil) and tranylcypromine (Parnate).

This next group are often mild anticholinergics. Physicians may prescribe them for dementia-related behaviors, but they should still be used in the smallest dose possible and should be monitored carefully.

- *Antipsychotics, atypical.* These second generation drugs are less problematic but still carry a black box warning. Although not approved by the Federal Drug Administration (FDA) for use with dementia, they are often prescribed for managing uncontrollable behaviors, even with LBD. Quetiapine (Seroquel) and clozapine (Clozaril) are the most commonly used, with varied results.

The following drugs are seldom used for dementia-related behaviors, but are often used by Persons living with dementia. These drugs can cause similar, but usually milder sensitivity symptoms, mainly because they tend to be both weaker and shorter acting:

- *Cold and allergy over-the-counter medications* containing antihistamines, decongestants and benzodiazepines. Examples: loratadine (Claritin), diphenhydramine (Benadryl) or chlorpheniramine (Chlor-Trimeton).

- *Opiates and other pain drugs* such as morphine or codeine.

- *Less safe ingredients* added to "safe" drugs. Examples: such as acetaminophen (Tylenol), aspirin or guaifenesin (Robitussin). These medications will usually have extra initials such as DM, CF or PM, which designate the additional ingredients.

The following behavioral drugs are less anticholinergic:

- *New antipsychotic:* Pimavanserin (Nuplazid) was FDA-approved in 2016 for use with psychosis in Parkinson's disease, a Lewy body disorder. Carries a black box warning. In the several online support groups that James follows, caregiver reports of drug effectiveness are mixed (par for the course with LBD!). However, he has not seen any reports of bad experiences. As new drugs often are, this drug is expensive, but low-income patients may be eligible for help with the cost, or with the higher co-pay.[5]

- *SSRI Antidepressants (Selective serotonin reuptake inhibitors). With* a low risk of sensitivity, these antidepressants are often prescribed for Persons experiencing depression and even for anxiety, but with limited success. They are more effective for the depressed care partner, but research has shown that the *use of antidepressants prior to age 65 is strongly correlated to a higher likelihood of eventual dementia.*[6] Examples: sertraline (Zoloft), fluoxetine (Prozac), paroxetine (Paxil) and escitalopram (Lexapro).

- **Dementia drugs.** These drugs were designed to improve cognition. They do not cure dementia, but besides improving cognition, they can help to manage many other dementia symptoms. Because of this, and because they usually have few side effects, one of these drugs may be the first "behavioral" drug the doctor prescribes. All of these drugs require live cells to work; as dementia kills the brain cells, they become less useful.

Donepezil (Aricept), rivastigmine (Exelon) and galantamine (Razadyne) are FDA approved to treat mild to moderate dementia. They act to preserve acetylcholine, thus limiting the damage done by Lewy bodies. With similar actions, they cannot be used together. Over the years, pharmaceutical companies have made improvements such as patches that decrease gastro-intestinal symptoms and extended release that allows smaller amounts of the drug to be metabolized over time. However, the basic formulas have not changed.

Memantine (Namenda) is FDA-approved for moderate to severe dementia. It has a different action than the above three and is often prescribed to improve their efficiency.

Drug Use in Care Facilities

Given the likelihood of sensitivities, choosing a care facility that uses as few behavior management drugs as possible should be at the top of one's list when considering placement of a loved one.

A facility's staff size is even more telling than their stated philosophy concerning behaviors and drugs. The more patients per staff, the greater the likelihood that the facility will resort to calming drugs. The number of staff often includes administrative staff and so even if the staff size appears good, it may not be.

The staff where my mom lives are caring and really seem to want to help her, but so often they seem to be short staffed and they can't spend the time with her that she needs. I visit and take up some of the slack, but I know it slips when I'm not there. – Marion, daughter of Rosalie

We've listened to many stories like Marion's from both care partners and staff. Care partners agree that most staff want to provide the best care they can. The physical care is usually good if staffing is adequate, but often it isn't.

Care facilities must operate at a profit and staff is their greatest expense. Cutting staff size is therefore the quickest way to economize. With decreased staff size, drugs are more likely to be used for behaviors than alternative options and care partners often complain that their directives concerning drugs are ignored.

Training is also important. Most states require staff to be trained in dementia care, but not for specific conditions like LBD, which may then be considered an unnecessary expense. Thus staff may not be trained in how to defuse the earlier appearing behavioral symptoms such as delusional combativeness before the behavior is so severe that drugs seem to be the only answer. Instead the facility may use more drugs or the Person living with LBD may be rejected as uncontrollable.

When considering long term care, ask if the facility:

- Has adequate care staff. This is the most important question you can ask. The smaller the staff, the greater the likelihood for overuse of behavior management drugs.

- Encourages staff to be accepting and positive.
- Teaches skills like empathetic listening and improv acting.
- Shows openness to trying new or different approaches to behavior management, i.e., those that may take more time and training but fewer drugs.
- Encourages staff to listen to and use care partner experiences and knowledge concerning their loved ones.
- Trains staff to use a variety of alternative options to deal with behaviors before considering drugs.

More Resources

The information in this chapter simply highlights the issues involved. The drug chapters in our earlier books have much more information about drug sensitivity and the drugs that can cause it. The Lewy Body Dementia Association offers a Medications Glossary, mentioned in the definitions at the first of this chapter. Download it and refer to it as needed!

***

Responsive Care Takeaways for Drugs and Sensitivity:

- Drug sensitivities, or overdose symptoms with a normal dose, occur due to a body's ineffective metabolization and waste management systems.
- Anticholinergic drugs limit the function of acetylcholine, a neuro-chemical that Lewy bodies also compromise, increasing the likelihood of drug sensitivity.
- Most behavior management drugs are anticholinergic, thus, alternative options for behavior management should be tried first.

- Small doses in combination with alternative options are less problematic and may be more effective than either alone.

- Some common over-the-counter medications considered safe by themselves are sometimes packaged in combination with extra ingredients that may trigger sensitivities.

- Sensitivities vary with people and drugs. Trial and error is the common way to discover what works best with each Person, although certain drugs are so likely to trigger sensitivities that they should be avoided.

- Responsive care involves a proactive interest in any prescribed or over-the-counter drug and a willingness to search out and try alternative options first.

- The smaller a facility's care staff, the greater likelihood of a dependence on behavior management drugs. A facility's biggest expense is staff. Expect to pay more for good care at a facility with low resident-to-staff ratios.

- The LBDA Medications Glossary and our books all offer much more information about drug sensitivity and the drugs that can cause it.

3. The Senses

senses: *Sight, smell, hearing, taste, and touch; faculties by which the brain receives external stimuli.*

attention deficit: *distractibility, impulsiveness, restlessness.*

selective attention: *Focusing on particular areas of sensory experience, rather than passively absorbing everything.*

over-stimulation: *More stimuli than the brain can process.*

nonverbal cues: *communication signals without the use of words—includes facial expressions, gestures, tone of voice, and other body movements.*

***

We actually have many different senses, but the main ones are sight, hearing, taste, smell and touch. The senses are the brain's information gathering system. Each sense sends the information it picks up to the brain via its own pathway. That is, something heard travels to the brain via a slightly different path than something seen or felt does. When any of these senses is damaged, the information delivered may be distorted or lacking.

Distorted or missing information. The normal brain uses a variety of skills to provide a more accurate perception. With limited access to these functions, the dementia-damaged brain takes the stimuli as delivered.

Dementia itself doesn't damage the senses. However, attention deficit, a common dementia symptom, limits one's ability to narrow one's focus and pay selective attention.[7] Everything gets equal billing, making it difficult to choose what to ignore and what to zero in on. This broader view sends fuzzier, less accurate information to the brain, even when the senses themselves are not damaged.

Language and the senses. Nonverbal cues are sensory messages learned as infants well before language skills, which require an extra decoding step in a different part of the brain. Thus, nonverbal cues remain easier to process than words, even for adults. When words and nonverbal cues picked up via the senses differ, humans in general tend to believe the more basic sensory cues over the words.

Language difficulties are a common early symptom for Persons living with LBD, but occur with other dementias as well. As they do, the Person will become dependent on nonverbal communication. They will become more alert for your nonverbal cues and use more nonverbal cues of their own to communicate needs and wishes.

Responsive caring involves learning how each sense works and the issues that might be involved. Learn to identify and accept the losses and then, to recognize the nonverbal cues used instead. This will help you to respond with a helpful attitude and action.

> ***Attitude:*** Patience is especially important as abilities slow and change.

> ***Attitude:*** Acceptance of the Person's abilities as they really are.

> ***Attitude:*** A willingness to work with the Person to help them use what is left to the best of their abilities.

Alternative pathways. Because each sense sends information to the brain via a different pathway, the senses are often used to circumvent dementia-caused problems and limit unwanted behaviors. Many alternative therapies, such music, aromatherapy and massage, use the senses in this way. Read more about these very helpful techniques in Chapter 26, Using the Senses.

Vision. It is normal with age for one's peripheral vision to narrow. Dementia may make this happen sooner. Thus as the dementia progresses, a Person with normal age-related peripheral vision will find their field of vision narrowing even more, so that it may be limited to a small area right in front of their face.

> **_Action:_** Stand in front of them, but off to one side a little so that you don't totally block their field of vision. (If you block it, they may feel threatened.)

The quality of vision also degenerates with age, other health issues, and possibly even with dementia. Things once clear can become blurry, faded and distorted. A Person may be sensitive to light and may appear to be sleeping when actually keeping their eyes closed as a way to maintain inner calm.

> **_Action:_** Use soft lighting and avoid dark shadows. Use strong, bright, contrasting colors to help the Person make better use of their remaining vision.[8]

Hearing. It is a common mistake for people to raise their voices when they perceive that they haven't been heard correctly. This doesn't work well with the Person--or with anyone else, for that matter. A louder voice is distorted and less easy to understand.

Gerry has been hard of hearing for years. I've learned that if I really want him to hear me, my best bet is to pitch my voice as low as I can and talk normally. When I shout, it triggers his anger and he can't hear me as well anyway. -- Olivia

Shouting is often equated with anger, triggering angry responses like Gerry's even in people who don't have dementia.

While dementia doesn't impair hearing, many people with dementia are of the age where being hard of hearing is common. Higher registers tend to be affected more than the lower ones.

Action: Use a normal voice, pitched as low as possible, to have the best chance to be understood.

Women's voices are normally higher-pitched than men's and anger often makes them shriller.

I hear women who use a low, deep voice better both literally and figuratively. Even if I can physically hear a high, shrill voice, it sounds unpleasant and triggers what Helen calls my "selective deafness." -- James, who wears hearing aids.

Like James, a Person may unconsciously block out an unpleasant sounding voice and the message will not be heard.

Unless some other problem has caused hearing damage, a Person with dementia will usually be able to hear no matter how far they are into their journey--and may be able to comprehend as well.

Action: Use care with what you say around a Person who appears to be inattentive or comatose. Inappropriate words can still cause agitation, inciting a new round of behaviors.

Attitude: Remain caring, loving and respectful even when you don't think a Person can hear or understand you.

Smell. All dementias affect the sense of smell eventually, but its loss can be an early symptom with Parkinson's disease and LBD.

Nathan hasn't been able to smell for years, not since he first started having Parkinson's symptoms. I'd like to use aromatherapy to help to calm him down sometimes because it is so easy to do but I wonder if it would help much since he can't smell. -- Elsie

Smell-based alternative options can still be helpful because odor receptors (olfactory nerves) reside in many areas of the body, including the skin.[9] Elsie should definitely try using aromatherapy with Nathan.

Touch. Touch is another long-lasting sense.

I notice that Nathan seems to touch things a lot more. And I have to watch him carefully because he'll put just about anything in his mouth. -- Elsie

Touch is most sensitive on the lips and tongue, fingers and palms, soles of feet and genitalia. Nathan is enjoying touching with these sensitive areas.

> ***Attitude:*** Show acceptance of any "odd" behavior due to tactile enjoyment. Monitor and protect so that the Person doesn't put unsafe things in their mouth. Showing your disapproval will likely cause anxiety...and other behaviors.

Persons also enjoy touching from others.

> ***Action:*** Touch often, using a gentle but firm hand. Avoid a light feathery touch that might cause unpleasant feelings of tickling or even "bugs."

As inhibitions decrease, some Persons can touch in sexually inappropriate ways for the same reason.

> ***Action:*** Set the scene so it isn't so likely to happen, like covering the genital area, and making sure friends know that his actions are not intentionally insulting.

Taste. Persons living with dementia often have altered food preferences with a loss of the ability to identify and remember tastes. Also, aging may cause the efficiency of the taste buds to fade. Thus a Person will tend to prefer sweets or other foods with strong tastes.

Nathan loves his sweets. But the doctor is talking to me about hospice. I wonder if a healthy diet matters that much anymore. -- Elsie

Care partners continually choose between pleasing their Person's ever-present sweet tooth and maintaining good physical health. The time eventually comes when enjoyment is more important than life-preserving choices.

Action: Sweets also make great bribe material!

Nathan still likes dinner time. He likes to sit at the table and have that bit of normalcy even if he doesn't eat much. I always try to have something to talk and laugh about. He doesn't say much, but he smiles and nods. -- Elsie

Even as the ability to identify tastes fades, the enjoyment of eating in general and the cultural processes around it lasts.

Attitude: Increase enjoyment by maintaining a calm and caring attitude. Mealtime is not the time for negativity.

***

Responsive Care Takeaways for the Senses:

- The brain's information gathering system consists of many types of senses.
- The five main senses are:
  o Sight, via the eyes
  o Smell, via the nose
  o Hearing, via the ears

40

- o Taste , via the taste buds in the mouth
- o Touch, via the skin
- Dementia seldom damages the senses but age and illness often does.
- Attention deficit, a common dementia symptom, limits one's ability to focus, resulting in:
  - o A broader view
  - o Fuzzier, less accurate information
- Persons living with dementia depend more on nonverbal cues as language gets more difficult to process.
- The senses provide alternative pathways to the brain that can be use by alternative therapies for changing behavior.
- Vision degenerates with age, becoming:
  - o Narrower
  - o Blurrier
  - o More sensitive to light
- Using a normal voice, pitched low, works better than shouting which may trigger fear responses.
- Smell-based alternative options can still be helpful even if the Person's sense of smell is gone.
- The sense of touch is long lasting.

  Actions:
  - o Be firm and gentle.
  - o Avoid an abrupt touch seen as "danger"
  - o Avoid a light touch which can be perceived as a tickle.
- Taste changes with age.
  - o Sweets remain favorites.
  - o Other strong flavors are also favorites.

4. Thinking Skills

dementia: *Significant impairment of least two cognitive functions.*

executive skills: *Used for judgment and reasoning, decision making and choices, organizing and sequencing, comparing and generalizing, connecting cause and effect.*

abstract thinking: *Uses executive skills to reason and develop concepts, including time-related ideas and levels of intensity.*

concrete thinking: *Primitive thinking based on material information derived from the senses in the here and now.*

showtime: *Appearing better than 'present normal' in the presence of a person other than the care partner.*

delusions: *Beliefs that aren't true, usually based on the first information the brain receives about an event or person.*

***

Dementia of any kind affects cognition, which includes memory and thinking. With Alzheimer's, memory tends to decline first although thinking abilities will also fade eventually. With LBD, thinking begins to fail before memory does. As thinking abilities fail, behaviors appear, thus they will appear earlier with LBD than they do with Alzheimer's or most other dementias.

Leon started thinking that people at the office "were out to get him." When he started yelling at customers, his boss told him he needed to get help. The doctor he went to referred him to a psychiatrist who, lucky for us, knew about Lewy. He said he didn't think it was a psychiatric illness but a neurological one. He diagnosed Leon with Lewy body dementia and recommended a medical retirement. -- Carla

What appears to be irrational behavior is often a rational response to an irrational belief. Leon felt threatened by the delusions his sick brain provided concerning co-workers and customers. His rational response was to protect himself. Angry displays and yelling were still inappropriate but impulsiveness is also a dementia symptom.

Leon's boss, co-workers and wife all tried to guide him back to rational thinking, so that the behavior would go away. Sadly, it doesn't work that way. Once a Person has a belief, it can't be changed. That takes abstract thinking, which is what dementia steals.

Children start with concrete thinking and as their brain develops, they gradually add abstract thinking. Good thinking is a balance of both; that's the norm for adults. However, abstract thinking requires executive skills, which fade as dementia progresses. As those skills fade, so does one's ability to think abstractly.

Of course, this doesn't happen overnight. Dementia progresses very slowly.

Nathan was a college professor and very smart. We didn't think much about it when his thinking got slower and he started forgetting a word now and then. He was in his seventies after all, and he was still smarter than most. Then he was diagnosed with Parkinson's and not long after that he began having hallucinations. He'd ask me if I could see what he did and if I couldn't, he'd nod and say, "Oh, hallucinations again, huh?" That was about the time he started worrying about me being stuck with an invalid. I'd tell him I'd rather be stuck with him, invalid or not, than anyone else and we'd be fine. -- Elsie

At first, thinking may simply be slow. With help, the proper connections can be made. Nathan welcomed Elsie's help as she supplied a forgotten word or explained that the child Nathan saw was a hallucination. He accepted her insistence that she didn't plan to desert him and believed her when she showed him that the scarf he'd thought stolen has simply fallen on the floor.

Then, the dementia progresses a little more.

He accuses me of planning to leave him, talking to my boyfriend on the phone, and all kinds of things like that. Oh, and he believes without a doubt that his hallucinations are real too. Worse, explaining and reassuring doesn't work anymore. The more I try, the angrier he gets. I'm so frustrated! -- Elsie

As with Elsie, it usually takes a while for a care partner to realize that what they did in the past is not working anymore, that what used to help is now making matters worse. When something fails, it is human nature to try the same thing over again, using a little more effort. Thus, Elsie's first response to Nathan's change was to try harder, with more emphasis and a louder voice. In turn, Nathan will misinterpret this increase in intensity as an attack and responded accordingly with increased behaviors.

Abstract Thinking

When a Person loses the ability to think abstractly, they lose the ability to develop ideas and concepts and to reason or make judgments.

Ideas. Ideas are mental constructs--plans, notions, desires, wishes, suggestions--generated from a thought or a collection of thoughts and are not, by themselves, abstract. They are however, the building blocks of concepts.

Concepts. Concepts are the finished product, evolved from a process that uses abstract thinking to fine-tune, prune and combine ideas with information from a wide variety of sources. As dementia develops, the Person loses the ability to use concepts to expand into things that aren't material, such as:

Time: A way of ordering events from the past through the present and into the future, as in: "I'll be ready to leave in 15 minutes."

> *Attitude:* Patience is the word! Patience when the Person wants to get ready right now for tomorrow's event or when it takes them ever so long to use the toilet or....

> *Action:* Use a timer to help your Person know when short amounts of time have passed.

Money: A way of measuring and comparing the value of services or items, as in: "My hourly wage is enough to buy this shirt."

> *Attitude:* Continue to recognize the Person as an adult even as you take over financial jobs that were once theirs.

> *Action:* Handling money is a sign of adulthood. Allow the Person to keep a few dollars in their pocket.

Possibilities: The "what ifs" of life, the likelihood that something might exist, as in: "I might win the lottery."

> *Action:* Use direct language, without modifiers like "if" or "when." These no longer mean anything to the Person.

Generalizing: To take something specific and apply it broadly, as in expecting the Person to sit quietly because you are sitting quietly, or because they did so in the past.

> *Action:* Expect to explain and direct each time. Be literal; avoid stereotypes.

Comparing: To estimate, measure or note the similarity or contrast between two or more things, as in: "This dress is too formal to wear to a picnic." (This statement also includes generalizations about formal and picnic wear.)

> *Action:* Talk only about one thing at a time—and keep it positive. Negatives get lost. "You would look good in this outfit."

Reasoning. Reasoning is the process of using abstract concepts such as comparison, generalization and possibilities along with physical evidence to think about something. Reasoning often concludes with a judgment.

Judgment. Judgment is the forming of an opinion or decision, using reasoning to weigh the validity of various ideas, concepts and physical evidence before coming to a conclusion.

> *Attitude:* Accept that reasoning and judgment are skills that require so much abstract thinking that they become lost arts early on.

Concrete Thinking

Dementia doesn't take away all of a Person's ability to think. Concrete thinking remains as abstract thinking fades. In fact, it lasts far into the journey, often to the end. Abstract thinking is important but we need concrete thinking too. It provides the specifics upon which to build the concepts of abstract thinking. When people become too abstract, they lose clarity.

Politicians are good at being abstract--at saying a lot without saying much at all! It's like the difference between "I plan to protect you" and "I put locks on the door."

However, concrete thinking alone limits one to those same specifics. Without the ability to think abstractly, the Person is left with only the basic information derived from the senses in the moment.

Concrete thinking requires a care partner's acceptance. It does no good to expect the Person to be able to think abstractly when they no longer can.

A Person doesn't lose the ability to think abstractly all at once. Their ability levels will also fluctuate. This is especially true for a Person living with LBD. If you practice being flexible and aware, you will be able recognize periods of higher abilities where you can relate with the Person a more complex level. You will also be more aware of their return to a lower level and able to adjust your own expectations and responses to fit.

Concrete thinking:

Is literal: Idioms and generalities no longer mean what they formerly did. A "hot potato" is just a very warm vegetable.

> *Action:* Be careful that what you say is actually what you mean. "That dress looks really good." not "That dress looks crazy hot."

Is in the here and now. There is no concept of past or present, no ability to wait, be patient or accept delayed gratification.

Action: Talk in the present, not the past or the future. "Let's go." not "If we leave now, we can get home in time to watch your video."

Is about instant gratification. Without the ability to see the value of future benefits, now is all that counts. A spoonful of ice cream now is better than the promise of a whole bowlful later.

Action: Use as a distraction or bribe. Bribes can backfire as a child learns to manipulate. But dementia decreases the ability to learn or even remember, thus the bribe serves as a distraction with no down-side.

Is single-minded. Focuses on only one issue at a time. This can and often does lead to obsession. Choices, comparisons and generalizations all require the ability to focus on multiple items.

Action: Talk about only one thing at a time. Avoid comparisons and generalizations and offer no more than two choices. "Do you want to wear this blue shirt or this red shirt?"

Is obsessional. Has difficulty dropping a highly charged subject such as a delusional belief in a care partner's infidelity. Letting go of an obsession requires the ability to consider other options.

Action: Use distraction, deflection and bribes to get the Person to change their focus and thus, let go of their obsession, at least for the moment. With LBD, memory may still be intact, and so they may return to an obsession later.

Is based on the FIRST information received about an event.

From the balcony of our hotel, Annie saw carnival lights in the distance and thought it was a fire. When I couldn't convince her that it wasn't, I pulled her back into the room. Then I asked her to help me unpack and she forgot about the fire. -- James

Annie saw lights and her brain's first judgment was "fire" which triggered her residual fear. The fact that the fear was from past experiences didn't matter. James's efforts to explain failed because she was stuck with her first piece of information..."scary fire!"

> *Action:* Use the Person's short attention span and distraction to help them move away from the fearful subject.

Is inflexible. Once something is decided upon, that's the way it is; there is only "what is," not "what might be."

> *Action:* It is futile to try to change a Person's mind. Instead, align with the residual feeling, join the person's reality and move the action along "It does look scary, doesn't it? Let's move away from here."

Is impulsive. Without the ability to see cause and effect, there is no consideration of future consequences. If the thought arises, the action follows.

> *Action:* Refuse to be upset by inappropriate words or actions. Distract and deflect instead.

Lacks empathy. Without the ability to consider other ways of seeing an event or to put oneself in the other's place, it's all about "me."

I told Nathan how hurt I was that he didn't trust me after all these years but he didn't seem to care. -- Elsie

Nathan wasn't trying to hurt Elsie or get even with her. He simply couldn't see anyone's pain but his own.

Attitude: Accept that the Person is not able to see how their behavior or words affect you.

Is two-dimensional, black and white. There are no gray areas, no almosts, no maybes. Something is or it isn't. There are no what ifs, or conditional situations. Emotions are either present or not present. There's no concept of level of intensity.

Action: Avoid conditional statements. The Person can understand "Let's play cards" much better than "If I clear off the table, we can play cards."

Is either apathetic or overly emotional. Apathy is a common dementia symptom. However, when emotions are present, they are likely to be intense no matter the provocation; that is the Person's only level.

Action: Look for other clues to the cause for distress or behaviors besides intensity.

Is closely connected to emotions, which aren't material, but can be felt. Unlike thinking, emotions remain.

Action: Take careful notice of emotions, both yours and the Person's, and focus on pleasant experiences.

The above changes in thinking change the way a Person sees their world, the way they interact with it and how they interact with you. Since the Person is stuck with their beliefs, you must be one who adjusts.

Action: Learn skills for dealing with concrete thinking without triggering behaviors. (Section Three)

Is more likely to be negative than positive. Humans are designed to pay attention to the negative warning messages before we do the more relaxing positive messages.

> *Action:* Learn skills for dealing with negative feelings and fostering positive feelings. (Chapter 15, Being Positive)

Delusions

delusions: *Dramas invented by the brain to make sense of sensory input when abstract thinking isn't available, which are often strengthened by residual emotions.*

residual emotions: *Emotions, often negative, left over from a previous experience.*

A delusion is a thinking disorder as well as a very troublesome behavior. It occurs when abstract thinking isn't available to process information gathered by the senses. Because thinking begins to fail early with LBD, delusions tend to appear early as well. They also appear with other dementias but usually not until much later in the journey. As abstract thinking becomes unable to test, evaluate and adjust information gathered by the senses, the brain invents delusional reasons for this information using whatever information it has available.

The Person is stuck with this interpretation of events. Delusions are "hard wired." That is, they cannot be corrected. Explaining, arguing or defending serves only to increase the Person's agitation.

> *Action:* Consider delusions unchangeable and go with them instead of trying to change the Person's reality.

Delusions can take many forms.

Story delusions. Some delusions are expressed as stories, often grandiose, triggered by something seen or heard and fueled by residual emotions around a dream, wish or other strong thought.

I went on a fishing charter in Alaska. You should have seen the fish I caught! -- Jack, a Person living with dementia

Jack has never been to Alaska but had always wanted to go there and go halibut fishing. His brain responded to the strong residual emotions attached to his wishes by perceiving them as reality.

Accusative delusions. Some delusions are expressed as accusations, usually triggered by fear or feelings of loss.

When I go to the grocery store, Nathan accuses me of having an affair with the clerk. I'm seventy! I wish I had that kind of energy. -- Elsie

Nathan's delusion is likely based on the already present (residual) fear he has of abandonment, which was the first information his brain received about Elsie's absence. The verdict is in and he will not be able to accept anything she says in her defense.

Mom is always accusing the staff of stealing her stuff when she's just mislaid it. -- Arlene, daughter of Clara

Arlene's mom's delusion is likely based on the continual feelings of loss caused by her dementia.

Misidentification. Some delusions are expressed as misidentification. Capgras Syndrome is the belief that a familiar person or pet has been replaced by a duplicate or impostor. A location delusion is similar. It is the belief about a familiar place or object being a substitute for the real one.

My mother would become very upset and insist that I was an impostor, and want to know what I'd done with her daughter. Nothing I'd say could convince her that I was really me. -- Arlene, daughter of Clara

Capgras and reduplicative par-amnesia are both signature Lewy body symptoms due to misinformation sent by the visual cortex. Like all delusions, they are hard-wired and unchangeable. However, because they are based on visual information, a Person can sometimes be reoriented by using others senses.

Paranoia: Some delusions are based on an irrational fear of something or someone.

When Brian sees an aide wearing red, he becomes combative. He is absolutely certain that staff who wear red are planning to cause him harm. -- Molly

As thinking fades, emotions become more important, with negative ones like fear being stronger. It is an easy step from that to attaching a delusional fear to something or someone, or in Brian's case, to the color red.

Fear is such a strong emotion that it can sometimes override abstract thinking. Even a person without dementia, or with only mild dementia, can be paranoid.

Fluctuating Cognition

Fluctuating cognition, a symptom unique to LBD, is when the Person's mind is temporarily much clearer at some times than it is at others. Clarity is most likely when the Person is rested and stress-free.

This transient clarity can provide the Person with more alertness so that during these times, they can be more independent and do more of their own care and even think more clearly.

> *Action:* Choose times when clarity is most likely for the Person's self-care tasks so as to increase positive feelings of self-worth, and decrease staff workload.

> *Action:* Use times of clarity to discuss any upcoming changes. The Person may not remember later but the emotional memory remains, decreasing the likelihood of behaviors.

During such times of alertness, a care partner and their loved one can enjoy togetherness "like old times," as described in this poem by Lynn D.[10]

An Old Flame
Yesterday I had a chance encounter
with an old flame.
He was every bit as charming as I remember,
and I was so glad to see him.
We had dinner together and talked
about everything and nothing at all.
It made me feel young again
and yes, I even flirted a little.
It was just so nice
to spend an evening being "normal".
I don't recall exactly when he left.
I just looked up and Charles was gone.
Lewy had returned.

Times of clarity can also lead to depression, when the Person sees too clearly their own plight and that of the care partner.

I've come to dread Carol's times of clarity because she sees all too clearly just what our lives have become and she's liable to start crying and begging me to just put her out of her misery.. -- Harold

This situational depression will likely disappear when Carol's clarity does. Lots of affection and reassurance will help too.

Showtime

Showtime is a special type of cognitive fluctuation well-known to most LBD care partners, although seldom documented in professional literature.[11] This temporary alertness, which tends to appear in the presence of someone other than the regular care partner can hide Behaviors and needs from doctors, visiting relatives or others who need to know the real situation.

At our last doctor's visit, the doctor asked Don to stand and I was so surprised when he jumped up like he was 18! Then the doctor told him to sit and stand a couple more times and Don kept on doing it easily. I feel like I've been played! -- Darlene

Don wasn't being manipulative. Showtime is beyond his control. It happens in reaction to a very normal impulse. We all like to be the best that we can be in the presence of people who are important to us. The difference is that we can recognize when it isn't worth the effort or is counterproductive. The Person cannot. When they feel the urge, they will make the effort. Showtime is also very tiring. Don probably slept most of the next day.

Showtime can last for a few moments or even several days. These longer episodes can be devastating when they end because they encourage the hope that the Person has been miraculously cured. They can also cause problems with care agencies.

We had Gordon evaluated for VA help but the social worker said he was too functional to meet their criteria. I explained that this was a "good day" and that he was usually not nearly this coherent, but she said she had to go with what she saw. -- Virginia

> ***Action:*** Keep a journal of the Person's behaviors that might help to make a more accurate evaluation, guide a doctor's decisions or help a distant loved one to better understand the Person's daily behavior.

***

Responsive Care Takeaways for Thinking Skills:

- Abstract thinking fades. It uses executive skills to reason and make judgments, is flexible and changeable.

  Attitude: Accept that the care person is the one who must change.

- Remaining concrete thinking uses current information from the senses and emotions to make decisions. It is literal, unconditional, single-minded and inflexible.

  Attitude: Let go of the expectation that the Person can change or understand idioms, concepts or levels of intensity.

- Concrete thinking is based on the first information available about an event, which is often an emotion.

  Action: When thinking is irrational, look for a residual emotion connected to the event.

- Delusions are dramas made up from what a Person with only concrete thinking perceives and feels.

  Attitude: Accept that delusions are hard-wired and flow with them instead of fighting them.

- Capgras Syndrome is a visual misidentification delusion.

  Action: To reorient, remove visual input and use a different sense, such as hearing, for communication.

- Fluctuating cognition, common to LBD degenerates gradually, but with highs and lows that can be deceiving.

  Attitude: Enjoy the "good times" of clarity but don't get caught thinking the dementia symptoms are really gone.

- Showtime is when a Person has a period of clarity with someone other than their regular care partner.

  Action: Keep a regular record to provide them with a better view of the disease's progress.

5. Perceptual Dysfunctions

perception: *A mental impression of what is sensed.*

illusion: *A perception of something real as something else.*

hallucination: *A perception of something that isn't really there.*

***

Perception is an ongoing two-step process. The brain uses:

- *selective attention* to sort out various sources of sensory input, ignore unimportant cues and collect those important for the task at hand.

- *abstract thinking* to compare this information to past knowledge, identify what is perceived, and locate it in time and space.

Perceptual dysfunction is an area where responsive caring works especially well. When a Person's perceptions are not the same as the care partner's, being able to recognize this, accept it and respond properly is much less stressful for everyone involved.

When senses begin to fail, we use selective attention and abstract thinking to compensate. However without the ability to filter or think abstractly, the Person must use the input from their senses "as is" to develop perceptions.

A Person with dementia may have perfectly functional senses: good eyesight, good hearing, etc., but have confused perceptions.

Annie stumbled and bumped into furniture a lot. We got her new glasses but she still stumbled. We went to a different optometrist--and then a third one, but nothing helped. -- James

Annie had a common dementia symptom, poor depth perception. Even though her sight tested well, her limited abstract thinking led her to misjudge where she was in relation to the furniture and caused her to stumble and bump into things. Her vision wasn't the problem--her muddled brain was.

The brain processes information from the senses in the cortex specific to that sense: visual (seeing), auditory (hearing), olfactory (smell), gustatory (taste) or somesthetic (touch). Although dementia may damage any or all cortexes eventually, the visual cortex is the one that tends to become damaged first. This is especially true for the Person living with LBD. However, there is hope. Even if a person had difficulty processing one sense they may be able to process another just fine. Thus, as vision becomes undependable, hearing or touch processing may still work well.

Illusions and hallucinations

Annie's brain might also have interpreted what she saw as being something else--an illusion. Illusions are most common with smaller items. A book on the floor is a dog, or a spot on the book is a bug. Perceptions can also become really wild, reporting that there's something there when nothing is that at all! These are hallucinations.

Annie would see a woman sitting on the sofa when there was no one there. Since the woman didn't seem to bother her, I said we could just leave her alone and let her rest. That seemed to satisfy Annie. -- James

Annie's brain was sending a false perception--a hallucination. Most hallucinations and illusions are benign. That is, they tend to bother the care partner more than the patient. With these, accepting and ignoring it, as James did usually works well. However, some hallucinations can be frightening or irritating. Find information about dealing with these more difficult hallucinations in Section Three.

Annie also heard phones and doorbells ringing. I'd answer the phone or the doorbell, but no one was ever there. -- James

Hallucinations can involve any of the senses, with visual being the most common, followed by audio. It's not unusual for a Person to experience bad "smells," even when their sense of smell has been gone for years. A Person might also experience a "bad taste" although this isn't common, or feel a "touch" usually from someone who seems to be just out of peripheral vision.

A person living with Parkinson's disease may begin to have failing visual perceptions well before their thinking fails.

I see little army men once in a while. They don't bother me. In fact they are sort of fascinating even if they aren't real. -- Brian

I have a little dog that follows me around. I call him Spot. I know he is an illusion, just something my mind makes out of a shadow or something, but he's company for me. And I don't even have to feed him! -- Ed

As their disorders advance into PD with dementia Brian and Ed will eventually lose the ability to think abstractly. Then they will begin to believe their hallucinations and illusions are real. This tends to happen within three years of when the hallucinations start.[12] This causes an understandable problem for the care partner who was used to being able to explain the hallucinations away. With responsive care, where information takes the place of denial, a care partner will be more able to recognize the change, accept it quickly and adjust their own responses to be more effective.

Misidentification

Capgras Syndrome is where the Person sees their care partner or other close person or even a pet as an impostor, a duplicate of the "real" person or pet. As with all delusions, the Person believes that their inaccurate perception is true and believes it completely. However, Capgras appears to be based on facial recognition cues.

Leon would look right at me and tell me I was an impostor. I insisted I wasn't and even asked him if I sounded like an impostor. "No," he said, "but you are. You don't look right." -- Carla

Vision is the sense that we as humans tend to use and believe first. If a person sees and hears conflicting information, they will believe their sight before their ears. Thus Leon believes his visual perceptions and discounts his auditory ones.

When I talk to her on the phone, Georgia knows exactly who I am. But when I'm in the room with her, she is often confused and thinks I'm that "other man." -- Frank

Frank might try speaking before he enters the room so that the audio recognition of his voice can trigger a recognition of him instead of the doppelganger.

When I crawled into bed last night, Don told me, "I don't think you should do that. What if Darlene finds out?" I was tired and so I just sighed, got in and turned out the light. I knew he wouldn't fuss; he never does." -- Darlene

Darlene didn't "look" like his wife, but she still felt like her and so with the lights out, he accepted her as such. This may not always work. Visual cues tend to trump other sensual cues unless the other cues are first so that they set the scene.

A location delusion is the belief that one's home, a familiar location or an object is a duplicate for the "real" one.

Brian tells me, "You can't fool me. This isn't my home. I know it looks like it but it isn't. I can tell. How did you make this happen? Where are we? Why are we here? I want to go home." -- Molly

Like Capgras, location delusions are visual perceptual dysfunctions. Therefore, try resetting the senses by taking the Person out of the area and bringing them back. This alone may do the job. If you can add some familiar incense and music while the Person is gone, this may hook other senses and increase your chance of success.

***

Responsive Care Takeaways for Perceptual Dysfunctions:

- Inaccurate perceptions combined with concrete thinking, can lead to delusions, followed by frustration at not being understood or accepted, followed by behaviors.

    Action: Be alert for changes in abilities so that you can adjust your own responses to be more effective.

- A person may have functional senses but confused perceptions.

    Action: When senses test out well, look for other reasons for the misperceptions.

- Hallucinations can involve any of the senses although visual is the most common. This is especially true for Person living with LBD.

  Action: View early visual hallucinations as a likely sign of LBD rather than Alzheimer's.

- People with Parkinson's disease may have hallucinations before abstract thinking fades and know at first that the hallucinations are not real.

  Action: View this as a warning sign that dementia is likely within three years.

- The brain processes each sense via a separate pathway. Perceptual processing may fail in one pathway before it does in another.

  Action: If information received by one sense is misjudged, try communicating via another sense.

- Misidentification delusions like Capgras Syndrome are visual malfunctions.

  Action: Use auditory or touch cues to reorient.

- Information delivered via the visual pathway is accepted as fact first.

  Action: Make sure the Person can't see you before trying to reorient with a different sense.

6. Emotions

emotions: *Feelings such as happiness, love, fear, anger. Can be triggered by situations or people or be residual.*

negative emotions: *motivators such as fear, anger and frustration that trigger behaviors.*

positive emotions: *feelings such as happiness and comfort that calm and relax.*

residual emotions: *Those left over in the brain from a previous experience.*

***

Emotions drive behavior. Humans relax or run away, depending on the emotions involved and how we choose to respond to them. However, we need abstract thinking to be able to make that choice.

In the brain, messages from the senses stop by the emotional center for an emotional charge, or reaction, before getting to the thinking center, where abstract thinking can do its job. If abstract thinking is limited or absent, these unedited emotions take its place and rule!

Negative emotions are motivators. They cause the body to secrete "fight or flight," stress-increasing hormones. They are intense, drawing and holding one's attention, pressing for change and movement away from whatever is causing the perceived discomfort. Negative emotions can be very stressful.

With Mason, his negative feeling is usually anger. He isn't a little bothered, or irritated, he's really angry, really focused on whatever the subject of the day is--it changes all the time! Sometimes, it's how I'm deceiving him. Sometimes, it's how the food is poisoned. Sometimes it's just that he hates having dementia! But whatever it is, he can't think of anything else and he gets almost sick because it is so stressful for him. -- Iris

Mason's concrete thinking prevents him from feeling gradients of anger. He is either not angry or very angry, and thus quite stressed.

Besides anger, some of the negative emotions common to Persons living with dementia are fear, frustration, anxiety, shame, grief, sorrow, discomfort, irritation, powerlessness, helplessness, ineffectiveness and guilt.

Positive emotions are comforters. They cause the body to secrete "feel good," stress-reducing hormones. These emotions are centering, relaxing, calming and seldom intense, which helps a Person stay comfortable. Positive emotions tend to relieve stress.

Some positive emotions common to Persons living with dementia are happiness, joy, pleasure, amusement, affection, love, friendliness, hope, relief, relaxation, serenity, calmness and satisfaction.

The strongest emotion rules. Milder positive emotions can seldom compete with the loud brash negative ones, especially where there is little abstract thinking for comparisons or evaluations. Whichever emotion is the strongest at the time is the one that rules. Thus, dealing with them is usually a two-part process: decrease the negatives and then add the positives.

If Mason is upset, I've learned that I can't get anywhere with him unless I deal with his anger first. I've found that if I nod and agree with him, he'll calm down enough that I can usually distract him with a treat. -- Iris

If Iris had tried to distract Mason with the treat before she defused his anger, his negative feelings would have still been in charge and he'd have brushed her off. When she validated his anger, Mason was able to let it go and respond to the positive feelings brought about by the offered treat.

Aligning with strong emotions by expressing a similar (but milder, so as not to escalate the issue) anger directed at the object of the Person's anger before moving on promotes a "we're in this together" feeling.

Emotions are remembered. Emotions are like the senses. They stay functional to the end. There's also an emotional memory that lasts long after dementia has eroded cognitive memory. These residual emotions color how we react to anything new.

For example, a man who had a wonderful time at a variety show may have a residual expectation that all variety shows will be fun. Likewise, a woman bitten by a dog as a child may have a residual fear of dogs. When someone with the ability to think abstractly meets a dog, they will have an initial fear, but then they can decide if the dog is safe or not. When a Person with only concrete thinking meets the dog, residual emotions rule and fear remains.

Residual emotions can be positive as well, like the memory of the fun time at the variety show.

Mason and I talked early on about residential care. We agreed about the reasons we might have to make that change and the kind of place he wanted to be in if that time ever did come. When it did, Nathan didn't remember our talks, but he didn't fight the move like I was afraid he would. -- Iris

A full participant in the earlier discussions, Nathan felt in control of his life when he agreed that he might eventually need residential care. The residual memory of his positive feelings of control and agreement helped him to accept the present situation.

Put simply, these facts are major tools for responsive care-- and for stress management:

- Negative emotions are strong and lasting.
- Positive emotions are mild and healing.
- Emotions last and are remembered.
- Residual emotions affect a Person's initial responses.

***

Responsive Care Takeaways for Emotions:

- Everyone has an initial emotional response to an event.
- Abstract thinking is used to evaluate and change one's initial emotional response as needed.
- Without abstract thinking, the emotions connected to the initial response drive a Person's behavior.
- Negative feelings:
  o Are strong and intense.
  o Motivate action.
  o Increase dementia-related behaviors.
- Positive feelings:
  o Are less intense.
  o .Encourage relaxation.
  o Decrease dementia-related behaviors.

- A Person's negative feelings must be dealt with before positive feelings will be effective.
- Emotions:
  - Can are triggered by immediate events.
  - Can become residual, left over from a previous experience.
- Emotional memory (residual emotion) lasts after cognitive memory fails.
- Residual emotions:
  - Can affect how *anyone* responds initially.
  - Become the Person's "truth" when abstract thinking isn't available for review and change as needed.

Actions:

- Avoid or remove anything that might cause negative emotions.
- Preserve or bring about situations that might cause positive emotions.
- Defuse negative emotions before offering positive experiences.
- Look for and respond to residual feelings that may be triggering behaviors.

7. Impulses and Disinhibition

impulsivity: *Acting without thought.*

delayed gratification: *The ability to resist an immediate reward and wait for a later, often larger or better one.*

disinhibition: *Acting upon an impulse, urge or temptation without considering consequences or social conventions.*

***

As the ability to control one's impulses or delay gratification disappears, everything is in the moment. When a Person feels a need to act, they act. They act without thought of consequences or other choices. Consequences are in the future and far too abstract. So is the idea that there might be a more appropriate time or place for an action.

My father went for a walk around the block. When I finally found him, he'd taken off all his clothes. I tried to get him to put some back on but he got mad and told me he didn't need them. When I said it was embarrassing, he just ignored me. I was so relieved when we got home and I could get him out of sight! -- Ariel, daughter of Ralph

Ralph was hot and so he did what came naturally. He took his clothes off. He wasn't able to see that this behavior was inappropriate or to consider other more appropriate choices.

Ralph couldn't understand what the fuss was about and so Ariel's complaints just made the situation worse. It wouldn't do any good to ask him not to do it again either. Because the behavior was an impulsive response to his discomfort, his brain wouldn't get past that and her request would be lost.

Complaints and requests for change trigger confusion and frustration. Bribes, which trigger positive feelings, work better.

Dad got out again but thank goodness, I caught him before he stripped. This time I just shrugged to myself and smiled at him. "Hey, Dad, I said. I was just going to have a dish of ice cream. Do you want one too?" Dad nodded and we went back into the house. It was so easy! -- Ariel, daughter of Ralph

When Ariel let go of her embarrassment and presented a calm, pleasant attitude, Ralph mirrored that and was able to respond to her ice cream bribe. By being pleasant, she didn't stir up angry emotions that would have kept him from accepting her offer.

Preventive planning, such as installing key locks on the doors can sometimes keep the behavior from becoming a problem. However, impulsive behavior is likely to happen at any time. Ariel can plan for this by making up apology cards, saying something like "Our apologies. This person has a brain disorder that may cause him to do odd things."

Dementia removes one's social filters, the need to be polite, for example, or think of what others might think, or even do.

We had visitors recently, people I knew but Walter didn't. They'd barely been seated when Walter spoke up and wanted to know when they were leaving. – Dee

Walter was not comfortable with people he didn't know and who were disrupting his normal routine. He impulsively said what he was thinking without a social filter.

Luckily my visitors were knowledgeable about dementia behaviors. They promised Walter they wouldn't stay long and

they didn't. Later, we went to dinner together without Walter.
– Dee

By doing her entertaining without Walter, Dee met her own needs while decreasing his distress.

Persons living with dementia can often say and do sexually inappropriate things. We are designed to find sex enjoyable. This doesn't necessarily change with dementia. However, we've been taught to keep sexual acts private. Dementia can change this. "If it feels good, do it," is the motto!

My mom was always a very proper person. Now she sits in her wheelchair in the nursing home hall and masturbates. The nurses don't stop her; they just take her back to her room where she can do it privately. – Marion, daughter of Rosalie

Marion's mom would not have considered doing such a private thing in public before she had dementia. The nurses are right not to try to correct her. She wouldn't understand the problem. Besides, if the activity entertains her, it can be beneficial. Of course, when done in public, it is embarrassing for others. The nurses addressed this by moving her out of the public eye.

I've just about stopped having my friends visit. I never know what Leon will do and even though I explain that he has dementia and doesn't understand what he's doing, they don't always understand. Once he walked up to my best friend and patted her breast. "You have great boobs," he told her. I wanted to fall through the floor. – Carla

Like Walter, Leon is simply saying what he is thinking without any concern for social appropriateness. Trudy is probably better off meeting her friends away from home, especially if they don't understand the reason for Leon's lack of social skills.

Responsive Care Takeaways for Impulses and Disinhibition:

- A Person acts without thinking of consequences, timing or appropriateness with unchangeable behavior.

  Attitude: Accept the unchangeable nature of this behavior.

  Actions:

  o Avoid complaints or requests that irritate.

  o Shrug, smile and use bribes to move your Person in the direction you want them to go.

  o Plan ways to prevent the behavior.

  o Use apology cards to help others understand that the Person's behavior isn't intentional.

  o Ignore inappropriate sexual behavior when not harmful but address the discomfort of others as needed.

8. Stress

stress: *Physical, mental or emotional pressure or tension*

stressor: *Anything that causes physical, mental or emotional discomfort or distress.*

stress threshold: *Amount of stress tolerated without damage.*

stress overload: *Amount of stress greater than one's threshold. Automatically considered a threat by the body.*

trigger: *Anything that causes stress overload and triggers a stress reaction.*

stress reaction: *The brain's automatic emotional and physical reaction to stress.*

fight or flight response: *The body's automatic physical response to a real or perceived threat.*

chronic stress: *Stress that lasts long past the immediate danger and is internalized as physical discomfort or damage.*

stress management: *Preventing, decreasing or removing stressors and being alert for triggers.*

***

The brain considers stress an emergency and diverts resources from other tasks to deal with it. This has a huge effect on dementia, and on most illnesses. It may not *cause* dementia but it uses up resources the body could otherwise use for resistance to such diseases—or for dealing with symptoms once a disease is present.[13]

Annie went into surgery with Mild Cognitive Impairment. She woke up with full-blown dementia. -- James

Annie's story shows how stress can speed up the advent of dementia. Surgery's physical assault to the body and the strong drugs required are both quite stressful. Many elderly people respond to surgery with temporary dementia (delirium). Most recover within a few days or at most, months. However, when Mild Cognitive Impairment, or any other LBD precursor such as Parkinson's or Active Dreams, is already present, a person may advance into true dementia as Annie did.

Responsive care works best if you understand how stress works and how to manage it. Stress is subjective. That is, something stressful for one person may be a fun challenge for someone else. What people call "stress" is actually excessive stress, or stress overload. We need a certain amount of physical, mental and emotional pressure (stress) to function and thrive, and then a little more for the challenge.

Everyone has a limit to the amount of pressure they can tolerate--a threshold. This threshold depends on the size of their reserves--resources left after regular needs are met.

> ***With dementia:*** Since the disease uses up much of a Person's resources, thresholds are usually already low and it doesn't take much more pressure to reach an overload.[14] "Stress" might come from something physical such as too much noise or being too tired. It might come from an illness such as a Urinary Tract Infection. Often, the stress will come from a misperception, such as a delusion.

Nathan's behavioral symptoms always get worse at the end of the day when he is most tired. I notice that they also get worse when he is feeling stressed by things like too many people or music that's too loud or even when I forget and don't talk slow enough. -- Elsie

When Nathan must use his reserves to deal with fatigue or stress, he doesn't have enough left to fuel his remaining abilities. He will be more confused and have even less impulse control.

The Stress Reaction

When anyone experiences more stress than they can tolerate, stress overload occurs, triggering a stress reaction. Triggers can be such things as feeling injured, overwhelmed, ill, tired, hungry, frightened, abandoned, insulted or anything perceived as a physical or emotional threat.

The initial response to such threats is to experience the "crisis emotions" of fear, frustration and/or anger. The job of these always negative feelings is to quickly instigate a "fight or flight" response.

> ***With dementia:*** These negative emotions drive a Person's behavior without being filtered by abstract thinking. Without the ability to judge how real or serious the "crisis" is, any situation perceived as stressful gets a full, vigorous response.

The negative emotions trigger the Autonomic Nervous System, which controls the body's voluntary functions, into action. It sends additional oxygenated blood (fuel) to organs required for a physical response[15] including:

The brain's perceptual centers. With increased awareness, one is better able to sense what's happening and respond quickly.

> ***With any dementia:*** Perceptions increase, while the ability to sort them out decreases, causing illusions and delusions. A narrowed focus makes more than one or two of anything confusing and overwhelming.

With LBD: Hallucinations and Active Dreams can already be present, often combining with poor perceptions of actual or imagined events to cause stress overload.

The circulatory and respiratory systems. Heart rate, blood pressure and breathing increase, so that more blood and oxygen can go to areas that need them for physical effort. The body is wired to react to a crisis physically even though most crises today are likely to be emotional. When there is little need for physical activity, the increased power appears as anxiety.

With any dementia: Anxiety increases a Person's already present negative emotions and increases the urgency to deal with any perceived stress.

The large muscles. Blood flows to the large muscles of the body so that a person can hit harder, lift higher, or run faster. When the muscles aren't used, this shows up as tension headaches, muscle cramps, lower back pain and similar symptoms.

With any dementia: The extra strength will usually show up as exaggerated movement such as swinging arms or a louder voice, and the danger of violence is greatly increased.

To provide all that extra power, the body decreases blood and oxygen to areas of the body that are less involved with fighting and fleeing, including:

The thinking centers of the brain. Taking time to think while being attacked by a saber-toothed tiger could get early man killed. He needed to rely on learned responses. The modern body is still not designed for thinking to be a crisis activity. With less oxygen, the brain gets fuzzy and slow, making tasks such as creative thinking and seeing associations difficult.

With any dementia: Even poorer than normal abstract thinking ability leaves the Person relying on crisis-generated negative emotions. Interpretation of these emotions becomes distorted and impulse control decreases. Change becomes a frightening series of new experiences.

With LBD: Communication may already be garbled and difficult. Stress will increase this.

The digestive system. Digestion is an ongoing process that can be sacrificed during times of crisis to provide extra energy for more needed functions. That's why a person may feel nauseous or constipated, or have diarrhea when frightened.

With any dementia: These responses are likely the same, but can be more damaging.

With LBD: Lewy bodies may begin attacking the digestive system well before any other symptoms are present, causing chronic constipation and other gastric symptoms. Stress may make any of these symptoms even worse.

The immune system. Immunity is a long-term process. It can be safely shut down for short periods, freeing up resources for more immediate battles. Shut down for long periods, it makes a person more susceptible to infections and other illnesses.

With any dementia: Even short-term stress can increase the likelihood of common dementia-related illnesses such as Urinary Tract Infections or pneumonia.

Care partner stress. Since the stress of caring for a Person living with dementia can cause "dementia-like symptoms" in care partners, they need to be as alert for these symptoms in themselves as in their loved ones. For example, a stressed-out care person's perceptions may be faulty and their thinking may be fuzzy. This can lead to negative behaviors that, when mirrored, increase the Person's already irrational behavior.

Long-Term Stress

When perceptions of threat continue over time, stress becomes internalized, greatly increasing the risk for illness— infection, dementia, heart problems, diabetes, cancer, etc. Stress does not *cause* these illnesses, but it does prevent the body from using all of its own resources to deal with them when they appear.[16]

With any dementia: Because Persons live day to day, long-term emotional stress is less likely.

With LBD: The Person's body is so compromised by the disease itself. This lowers their threshold so that even small amounts of stress can be problematic over time.

Care partners. Long-term stress is much more of an issue for care partners. They are especially susceptible to long-term stress, with all of the accompanying illnesses it can bring.

I have diabetes. When I'm stressed, my sugar levels shoot up and if I'm not careful, I can get really sick. Last summer, I ended up in the hospital and Mason had to go to a respite center. The doctor told me that if I didn't get help caring for Mason, I'd likely be back in the hospital again. -- Iris

While stress didn't cause Iris's diabetes, it hindered her body's ability to use its own resources to fend off the illness or deal with it when already present. Caregiver stress is a very serious issue. A care partner who does not practice safe self-care often dies before their loved one does.

Treating Stress

A medical doctor may treat stress by prescribing a relaxant for whatever is physically causing the stress. While one should always try to treat the cause, the physical reason isn't necessarily the real cause. For example, stressfully tight muscles can be relieved with drugs, but what caused the tight muscles in the first place? Muscle tightening is part of the fight or flight response to stress, which in our culture is likely something emotional.

A psychiatrist may prescribe an anti-anxiety or antipsychotic drug for emotional stress--and getting rid of emotional stress is a good thing to do. However, besides the fact that these drugs are likely to be Lewy-sensitive (See Chapter 2, Drugs and Drug Sensitivity), the emotional stress is still only a symptom or a response to the real cause.

A neurologist may prescribe a dementia drug to decrease LBD symptoms--including behaviors and other stressful symptoms. In many cases, this can be quite helpful, improving cognition and decreasing non-cognitive symptoms like hallucinations with few side effects. However, these drugs, not very powerful to start with, require live neurons to work. As the disorder progresses and kills off the neurons, dementia drugs gradually become ineffective. And like the previous drug groups, these treat the symptoms, not the true stressors.

Most alternative options for behavior management are aimed at preventing, decreasing or removing stressors. As with drugs, alternative options will not cure the dementia or even do away with all of the behaviors. However, these options can often manage the behaviors with more safety and a better quality of life than drugs alone can.

Alternative options are often used in combination with drugs, so as to have the advantages of both. The use of the alternative options makes it possible to use fewer drugs for the same effect and adds quality of life. Every person is different however. This is especially true when talking about Persons living with LBD. Some people are super-sensitive and are not able to tolerate any amount of drugs, even the small doses used with alternative options.

Responsive care involves:

- Understanding how real or perceived stress causes negative feelings and an urge to act.
- Learning what the Person's stressors are likely to be.
- Being alert for these stressors and their triggers.
- Monitoring one's own stress level and doing what is needed to keep it low.
- Working with the Person's medical team to put into action the safest and most efficient mix of behavior management options.
- Stress management drugs are recommended only after other options have been tried, and then in as small a dose as possible, preferably in combination with alternative, non-drug options.
- Alternative stress management tools will usually be a mix of prevention, empathy, acceptance and relaxation.

How It All Fits--or Fails--Together

The senses, perceptions, emotions and thinking centers all work together to gather, process and act on information. Then if the information is perceived as a threat, this is how the process works--or fails.

For example, Neil's father, Dan, has dementia, is hard of hearing and is known to have depth perception issues. Jane is a new staff person in the care center where Dan lives. She comes into his room and begins to help him move from his wheelchair to his bed. Jane talks to Dan, but her voice is high pitched.

- The senses gather the information. When any of them are damaged, the information may be inaccurate even before it reaches the brain.

Dan: This person doesn't look, smell or sound like anyone I know. Her voice is high and loud. She is standing very close to me and making sudden movements.

- The information travels to the perceptual center, where concrete thinking accepts it as is, without judgment, gradations or conditions.

Dan: This stranger that I don't know or trust sounds angry and is acting in a dangerous manner.

- Then the information passes by the brain's emotional center and triggers an emotion, often based on past experience. For the Person, these residual emotions can be powerful.

Dan: I'm scared. I feel threatened.

- Abstract thinking comes next, where the information, emotions and initial perceptions are reviewed and moderated. Without the ability to think abstractly, a Person is left with their initial perceptions turned into fact, charged with whatever emotion is strongest and a firm belief that this information is correct.

Dan: I am being threatened. This angry stranger is threatening to hurt me. I need to protect myself.

- Based on these conclusions, an action is chosen. Without the ability to contemplate consequences or make choices, the first action the Person considers is the only action considered.

Dan: I can hit out and drive her away. (Another Person's first solution might be to cry, or scream.)

- The action occurs. If the processing was limited or muddled and the emotions elicited were negative, the action is often a behavior.

Dan hits out at Jane.

Jane could have intervened at several places in this scenario. For starters, she could have:

- Used a softer, slower tone.

- Moved more slowly and explained her actions as she went.

- Used nonverbal cues, such as smiles and a gentle, firm touch.

- Asked Neil to come into the room with her at first, so that his father would feel safer with a familiar person there besides this stranger, Jane, that he didn't know and couldn't yet trust.

***

Responsive Care Takeaways for Stress:

- Stress uses up resources a person could otherwise use to resist or deal with diseases, including dementia.

- "Stress" is really excessive stress, more than a person can tolerate without damage.

- The brain responds to perceived stress by increasing oxygenated blood to:
  - Perceptual centers, increasing the likelihood of hallucinations or delusions.
  - Large muscles for increasing strength, and the likelihood and of muscle cramps and of the Person striking out at an imaginary foe.

- The brain borrows oxygen from these systems that aren't needed in an immediate physical crisis:
  o Thinking centers, resulting in poor decision making.
  o Digestive system, resulting in abdominal cramps.
  o Immune system, with increased chance of infections.
- Stress is often more of a problem for the care partner than for their Person because it can be longer lasting.
- Long-term stress internalizes and becomes a risk for illnesses.
- Extreme stress can express as temporary dementia with many of the same symptoms including irrational thinking.
- Drugs usually treat stress symptoms rather than removing the stressors.
- Alternative options for behaviors are aimed at preventing, decreasing or removing stressors.
- Alternative options used in combination with drugs may be quicker and more helpful than either alone.
- Responsive care involves being knowledgeable about stress, what it does to the individual Person, and finding the safest and most efficient way to manage it.

9. Mood Disorders

mood: *Emotional states that can last a long time. Longer lasting negative moods are often considered to be disorders.*

empathy: *An awareness of other people's emotions, a key element in the link between one's self and others.*

empathy deficit: *inability to feel empathy, which can appear as indifference or self-centeredness.*

apathy: *A lack of motivation and the inability to initiate.*

depression: *a persistent feeling of sadness and loss of interest in activities once enjoyed.*

symptomatic treatment: *That which affects only symptoms, but not the cause.*

***

Empathy deficit, apathy and depression are separate entities that often accompany dementia. Although they are caused by different brain dysfunctions, they have many similarities. All three:

- Are closely related to the Person's emotions, usually negative.
- Can occur often in dementia, especially LBD.
- Can show up alone or can accompany one or both of the others.
- Can show up as lack of interest.
- Are not something the Person can control or change.
- Can trigger negative emotions--sometimes in the care partner more than in the Person!

Treatment for all three is also similar:

- Treatment is mostly symptomatic only.

- Acceptance and validation is the primary requirement.
- Alternative options for relaxation, comfort and clarity.
- Dementia drugs may help since these can all be LBD-related symptoms.
- Mild antidepressants may help and are usually considered safe.

Empathy Deficit

Empathy is what people use to try to understand another's feelings. As thinking fades, emotional sensitivity increases and a Person becomes more aware of other's feelings. However, this doesn't mean they are more understanding. Emotional sensitivity and empathy are very different.

I had an argument with my daughter before I went to visit Joe in the nursing home. He picked up the anger I was still feeling and started accusing me of running around on him, calling me awful names and telling me to leave. -- Alice

Once Joe identified the feeling he picked up from Alice as anger, it became his own. His damaged brain found a residual fear of desertion that provided a reason for his anger. (Without the ability to comprehend "might" or "later", what he fears might happen in the future, HAS happened NOW in his mind.)

Empathy is a two-step process:[17]

- *Affective empathy,* where you feels another's emotions as though they were your own. You experience this when you see a friend's painful toe and your perfectly healthy toe twinges in sympathetic pain.
- *Cognitive empathy,* where you use abstract thinking to identify feelings as the other person's, and not your own. "She feels sad. I'd feel that way in her situation also."

Joe did affective empathy just fine. He picked up Alice's anger and felt it. The problem was that he couldn't take the next step and identify it as hers, not his. Dementia makes everything personal.

I started crying and asking why he was trying to hurt me. He just yelled more and said I was the one who was hurting him. I'm devastated. Joe was always such a gentle man and I used to be able to talk with him about anything and he'd understand and help me work through it. I miss that so! -- Alice

Once a man of great empathy and wisdom, Joe is now unable to provide either. With only concrete thinking, Joe could no more put himself in Alice's place and understand her pain than he could understand that his anger was really a reflection of hers.

Dementia keeps a Person in the present and makes everything personal. The concept of "I'd be angry, or sad, or hurt, *if* that happened to me" is just too abstract. One either is or isn't. An inability to feel cognitive empathy appears to be about twice as likely for people with early LBD than for a person with no dementia.[18] The likelihood is even greater in later stages.

With responsive caring, a care partner can choose to see their Person's uncaring attitude as a symptom of the disease. With this view, it is easier for you to avoid reacting out of pain or anger, hold onto resentments or to see their lack of empathy as a failure on your part. By recognizing the Person's reflected pain as real to them along with the resulting negative emotion, you can more easily validate the feeling and move on. To help others avoid being hurt or confused, consider preparing an apology card explaining that the Person has an illness that impairs their ability to understand the effect of their actions.

When the Person can no longer feel empathy, a connection is lost between them and the care partner, and there can be loneliness as well as loss. A support group of people going through similar experiences can be a great help. Hurt feelings can build up even though you know intellectually that the Person's indifference is beyond their control. A support group is an understanding and safe place to talk about your situation and the not always pleasant feelings involved.

Apathy

Apathy occurs when there isn't enough dopamine in one's system. Parkinson's families know dopamine as the neurotransmitter that controls mobility and one that Lewy bodies target and deplete. It is also one of the "feel good" chemicals in the body. When dopamine is low, apathy can appear, blunting both negative and positive feelings.

Steve used to be busy all the time. He was a great carpenter and built all of my kitchen cupboards. But now, he just doesn't seem to care much anymore. And he used to be really sensitive to my feelings too. Now he'll say awfully hurtful stuff sometimes and not even be aware of how it hurts me. Even if I tell him, he just shrugs. -- Rhonda

Steve's inertia and indifference is not intentional; it is just apathy showing up. Apathy is sometimes defined as "the lack of empathy."

I can sometimes get Steve interested in something easy like looking at the family photo album if I get it out, start leafing through the pages and talking about the photos. -- Rhonda

Rhonda was modeling the behavior she wanted Steve to mirror. He can't initiate, or get the album now himself, but he'll look at it if she does too.

I've learned to take my time and just focus on simple things. Everything is just so difficult for Steve now. -- Rhonda

Rhonda's patience is important. It is true that apathy blunts feelings in general, both negative and positive, but that's not all it does. Apathy damages the Person's ability to care about *anything*, start anything or even follow through once a project is started. It makes everything so much more difficult for the Person that it adds frustration and stress. This is especially true if it triggers negative feelings in their care partner as well.

Depression

Depression changes one's mood, thinking, physical well-being and behavior. It generates feelings of sadness, misery, unhappiness, anger, loss and frustration. These negative feelings in turn are likely to generate a variety of behaviors, such as anxiety, irritability and restlessness.[19]

Performing tasks, making decisions or interacting with others all become more difficult. Since these are also skills affected by dementia, depression makes them even worse.

Chronic (organic) depression can be caused at least partially by a lack of serotonin, one of the "feel good" chemicals. This type of depression, more common with LBD than with other dementias, can be quite long lasting. Situational depression is a response to an unwelcome life-change, such as a diagnosis of dementia. This type is usually short term. With time and possibly treatment, it can improve and eventually disappear.

Carol isn't apathetic. She is still willing to go out for ice cream and such. But she can get awfully sad. I've noticed that her thinking gets even slower then too. The bouts of depression often follow her periods of clarity. -- Harold

Nancy's depression is likely situational, brought on by the knowledge about her illness. Apathy and depression often appear together. When they do, the situation is more serious because motivation is affected as well as mood.

Be aware that ongoing situational depression is common with care partners. As a response to the continual bombardment of new responsibilities, new losses, feelings of inadequacies and not enough support or help, it can last a long time.

I just feel so overwhelmed all the time. I love Carter, but this is a very demanding job and I don't have much help. I've got so I don't want to do anything I don't have to do anymore--no, I can't do any more than I have to and even that's an effort! -- Gwen

Gwen is experiencing caregiver depression. If she doesn't get help quickly, her situation will get even worse as Carter picks up on her negative feelings and expresses them as behaviors.

Alternative therapies using essential oils may elevate moods. Other relaxing alternative options such as massage may also help.

***

Responsive Care Takeaways for Mood Disorders in General:

- Empathy deficit, apathy and depression can show up alone or together.
- All three can express as indifference.
- All three can be difficult to tell apart.

  Attitude: Don't worry about what causes these changes.

  Action: The care will be the same.

- These mood disorders are all symptom of the illness.
- The Person has no control over these mood disorder behaviors.

  Attitudes:

  o Acceptance that the behaviors are due to the illness, not the Person.

  o Lowered expectations, which decreases the Person's feelings of inadequacy, especially with apathy and depression.

  o Patience, which will decrease anxiety and the need to perform.

- Mild antidepressants, dementia drugs and a variety of alternative remedies may help to decrease symptoms.

  Attitudes:

  o An acceptance that treatment is symptomatic.

  o An understanding that treatment can also be very helpful in reducing behaviors.

Actions:

o Use communication skills, empathy and other alternative options to complement or sometimes to replace medical treatments.

o Use positive responses to decrease behaviors.

Self-care:

o Refuse to take the indifference or other behaviors personally.

o Monitor yourself carefully and have adequate help and support. Add more personal time as needed.

o Use a support group to relieve loneliness and as a safe place to vent hurt feelings.

***

Responsive Care Takeaways Specific to Empathy Deficit:

• Empathy is a two part process involving a) feeling another's emotions as though they were your own and b) identifying them as the other person's.

• A Person is an expert at picking up feelings but without abstract thinking, cannot identify them as anyone's but their own.

Action: Make a sincere effort to validate the Person's reflected, but still painful, feelings so that both of you can move on.

***

Responsive Care Takeaways Specific to Apathy:

- Apathy is caused by lack of dopamine, a pleasure hormone in the body (and a neurotransmitter that facilitates mobility).

- Apathy blunts feelings, resulting in a lack of motivation and an inability to initiate or care about anything.

  Attitude: Do not expect the Person to be able to recognize your feelings as yours or to understand them.

- A Person can mirror behaviors and follow actions long after they can initiate them or do them on their own.

  Action: Try modeling a behavior you want the Person to mirror or start an activity and invite the Person to join you.

***

Responsive Care Takeaways Specific to Depression:

- Depression is an ongoing sadness that interferes with life in general and makes everything less enjoyable, more tiring and more difficult.

  Attitude: Maintain a positive attitude so that the Person can mirror it and possibly, decrease their own sadness.

- Situational depression is caused by life-situations such as an unwanted diagnosis and is usually temporary.

  Attitude: Recognition that although temporary, situational depression is equally depressing.

- Chronic depression is at least partially caused by a lack of serotonin, a "feel good" chemical, and can be long-lasting.

95

- Chronic depression is more common with LBD than with other dementias.
- Exercise, social interactions, adequate sleep and a pleasing environment all work to decrease depression.
- Dementia drugs act to treat other disease-related symptoms including depression.
- Many non-drug remedies improve depression.
- Many depression drugs are considered safe to use with dementia.

Actions:

o Expect some improvement from cognition drugs that treat all LBD symptoms.
o If depression is still present, try non-drug remedies.
o If depression is still present, work with the physician to add low doses of the milder depression drugs.

Care partners are prone to situational depression which can become long-term, with negative feelings reflected back by the Person as behaviors.

Actions:

o Monitor your own moods and do good self-care so as to avoid caregiver depression.
o If caregiver depression is present, get help immediately.

Section Two: Putting the Care Partner First

self-care: *making sure one's ability to perform a necessary job is not damaged by neglect, overwork or emotional distress.*

martyrdom: *the act of putting someone else's needs first, at the expense of your own to the extent that it becomes damaging.*

Self-care is one of your most important behavioral management tools. A Person with a happy, healthy, unstressed care partner will also be happier and more content, with fewer behaviors. The converse is also true:

- When you are depressed and irritable, the Person will likely reflect these negative emotions, often as behaviors.
- When you are overburdened or stressed, you cannot deal as easily with present behaviors, which likely will then increase.

Responsive care is not just about the Person. If you don't take care of yourself, the Person will at best, have an inefficient, overburdened, often ill, often irritable care partner. You wouldn't accept that in a paid caregiver and you shouldn't accept it for yourself.

That doesn't mean that self-care is easy. It takes effort, determination and planning. Staff in care facilities can separate their work from their personal time because they go home after work. As a care partner, you are likely on the job 24/7. You must make a more conscious effort to identify some time as yours, to be used for your own needs. Self-care is not selfish, but necessary for the Person's best care.

If you are like most care partners, you understand intellectually that you need to take care of yourself but all too often this doesn't happen. As the Person's needs increase, you see these as more urgent than your own and slip into always putting them first. This martyr-like behavior can eventually make you dull, ineffective and even unsafe, like the carpenter's poorly maintained saw. There is also a greater risk of accidents such as falls and back strain, serious illnesses and even death.

You can change this by caring responsively for yourself:

- Start by recognizing your own value and viewing your needs as important and as necessary as your loved one's needs. Not only is your well-being an important behavior-management tool, it is also your loved one's *most important need.*

- The Person often has urgent needs. Accept that urgency doesn't mean important. Learn to prioritize and identify what can be left for later or not done at all.

- Make meeting your basic needs a priority.

- Don't try to do it all yourself. Find ways to share your load with others.

- Learn to be flexible, to let go of "what was" and accept "what is."

- Use improv acting to incorporate behavior management skills in an easy to understand and acceptable format.

- Take regular periods of respite, so that you can come back feeling refreshed and able to do a good job.

10. Basic Needs

As a human being, a care partner has certain needs that must be met to function well. These are actually the same as the ones for decreasing the risk of dementia:

- Stress management
- Adequate sleep, fluids
- Healthy diet
- Exercise
- Good medical care
- Spirituality
- Personal time and meditation
- Socialization

All are equally important and interconnected. For example, unmanaged stress can cause a lack of sleep or other problems with your basic needs, while how well you manage your stress depends on how well you take care of your other basic needs.

Start by recognizing your own value. You are the most important person in your Person's life and their most powerful dementia care tool. Don't underestimate your value! Until you place value on yourself, you won't pay adequate attention to your needs.

Stress can be a huge issue for the care partner. Care partners are especially at risk for long-term stress and all of its issues.

I think I'm getting dementia! I'm making crazy mistakes and forgetting far too much and yesterday, I flew off the handle with Nathan. I was so ashamed of myself later. I guess I really do need a break. -- Elsie

Most care partners have felt like Elsie at some time or another. Stress causes dementia-like symptoms--not dementia, but symptoms: cloudy, self-centered, sometimes irrational thinking, forgetfulness, anxiety and irritability. *A person with dementia symptoms taking care of a Person with actual dementia is a sure setup for failure.*

A Person living with dementia lives day to day. They don't carry around emotional stress the way a care partner may. However, because they mirror a care partner's emotions, they experience that stress second hand and reflect it back as behaviors, making more stress for the care partner. Illnesses and injuries may increase for both. Caregiver mortality increases. Yes, you may die, and then where will your loved one be? Care partner stress management is a primary aspect of dementia care.

Respect the value you have as the Person's connection to the rest of the world, as their physical and emotional caregiver, and their stability. Without you, their care can degenerate markedly.

Next recognize your limitations. You aren't superhuman; you can't do it all perfectly. You may not even be able to do it all imperfectly! You may get to the place where you can't do it period, if you don't ask for help. This is probably the biggest roadblock a care partner faces--a resistance to asking for help. Most care partners who finally do ask for help say they wish they'd done so sooner.

Then, take care of your physical, mental and emotional health. This means paying attention to your own basic needs.

Adequate sleep is a requirement that is often the most difficult to get.

Tony tossed and turned last night. He was having those active dreams again. Neither one of us got much rest. He slept in this morning and now he's napping. I could use a good nap too, but I like to use his nap times to do the things I can't do when he's awake and I'm at his beck and call. -- Angela

Tony's active dreams (REM sleep behavior disorder) are common LBD symptoms. Tony was asleep while he was dreaming and thrashing around, but it kept Angela awake. Many care partners end up moving to a separate bed or bedroom just so they can get the rest they need.

Carol woke up at two this morning and thought it was time to get up. I finally convinced her it wasn't and got her tucked back into bed. She went right back to sleep, but by then I was wide awake. It took me another hour to settle down. -- Harold

Carol's dementia-damaged sleep rhythms are off, waking her up at the wrong time. Having to be awake and alert during the night also disturbs Harold's sleep rhythms, especially if it is a common occurrence. He needs about seven hours of sleep a night on a regular basis to avoid experiencing those stress-related dementia symptoms!

Tony and Carol may be able to catch up on their sleep during the day. Care partners understandably want to use these nap times for things they can't do easily when the Person is awake. It might be a good time to consider a nap instead. The nap may not be as good as getting a good night's sleep in the first place, but it can stave off those symptoms of fatigue. Some care partners use the time when a helper is there during the day to nap. Others have their helpers come in at night, so that they can keep their normal sleep routine.

Adequate fluids can be easy to forget. You need about eight glasses of fluid (preferably water) a day to function well.

I'm extra careful to make sure Gerry gets enough to drink, but I forget about myself. I know I need to get those glasses of water in. When I don't, I get really tired and irritable. Sometimes, I even get muscle cramps. -- Olivia

Dehydration, like lack of sleep, can cause dementia-like symptoms. Make a habit of drinking a glass of water the first thing in the morning. (Add a few drops of lemon essential oil for a mildly lemony drink that helps to stave off infections and illnesses.)

Identify several other times during the day, such as before meals or during exercise where you can make drinking a glass of water a routine. When you offer water to the Person, join them with a glass of your own.

Healthy diet. A Mediterranean diet is considered the best, most nutritious diet not only for the Person, but also for care partners. It involves eating mostly plant-based foods-- whatever vegetables and fruits you like best--along with fish, whole grains and nuts.

I tend to eat on the run a lot, just make a quick sandwich, or something easy. And when I have a rough day, I love my comfort food--anything salty and starchy. Oh, and sweet, I keep sweets around for Gerry but find myself eating them up. -- Olivia

Care partners often find it difficult to maintain a healthy diet. If like Olivia, you eat on the run, make at least one mealtime a day a priority, a time where you sit at a table and eat a meal, with others or alone.

As for comfort foods, don't give them up entirely, because they do give you a psychological lift. However, physically, starchy foods tend to make you more tired. With that in mind, consciously choose fruit instead a cookie, or something else entirely such as playing games on the on the computer.

For more about diet and nutrition, see Chapter 11. The information there is as applicable to the care partner as it is to the Person.

Exercise, extremely important as a stress fighter, is not always easy for a home-bound care partner to get. All movement helps.

I'm actually pretty sedentary. I never did exercise much. But now that we are dealing with dementia and I'm usually feeling stressed, I see how important it is. Dad and I go walking every day and I usually come home feeling so much better. -- Ariel, daughter of Ralph

Whenever possible, develop a routine of exercising with the Person, making it an enjoyable together time. You still need any exercise you can get on your own as well. Go for walks, ride a bike or go to an exercise class. If you can't do that, do aerobics in front of the TV, chair exercises while at a computer or even stretches on the bed before you sleep or after you wake up.

Good medical care for yourself is a necessity. Be as diligent about getting this as you are for the Person. Don't put it off because you just don't have time or energy for "one more doctor's visit" or even the money. If you get seriously ill, the time, energy and cost will be much greater. Maintaining good health pays you back for the time it takes in improved energy and saved money.

Spirituality is very personal and tends to be different for everyone. Don't let your focus on caregiving cause you to drop your spiritual practices. These can provide inner strength, comfort, a feeling of connectedness with others and a sense of oneness with God or a higher power. There's research that shows that caregivers with a strong perception of spirituality have less depression and anxiety and experience a better quality of life. They tend to feel less burdened and are better able to handle stress.[20]

I don't know how people do this without God. He is my anchor and a vital support for my journey. When Gordon gets difficult, I stop, take a couple of deep breaths and say a short prayer. It really works. I can just feel the strength flow in and I can keep on doing what I need to do--and do it without losing my temper!--that's the wonderful part. -- Virginia

Pat Snyder, author of Treasures in the Darkness, tells the care partners in the classes that she teaches, "Whenever we are helping someone who is hurting and vulnerable, as those with dementia surely are, I call that God's work."

My faith changes the way I see my world. Instead of focusing on the drudgery and difficulties of our daily struggles, it helps me to see the value in my work. It isn't the drudgery of cleaning up Gerry's messes, it is the glory of showing love and concern. It isn't the embarrassment and pain of Gerry's accusations, it is the knowledge that God knows, and therefore I know, that I'm not the awful person his delusions tell him I am. -- Olivia

Make sure you continue to do whatever you've always done to maintain your spirituality. This doesn't necessarily mean going to church, synagogue or meetings, but being with others with similar beliefs can be a great help. If you've never been religious, remember spirituality takes many forms. Find one that works for you and put it into practice. BethIsreal Hospital offers an article that gives many suggestions about how care partners can identify, maintain and use their faith.[21]

Religious communities can also provide physical help. Many have programs where they will visit and give you a few hours away, do chores such as lawn mowing or bring food. Be sure to check this out.

Personal time is another basic need that often gets ignored. Make a conscious effort to regularly fit personal time into your routine, perhaps while the Person is napping or otherwise engaged.

Meditation, where you clear your mind and focus on nothing but your breathing is best done for at least five minutes at a time. There's good research that meditation can lower your stress for hours afterward. The relaxation exercises in Chapter 27 offer more information about ways to relax your mind and body.

Some care partners prefer to find a quiet place to read or do something creative or fun. The main thing is to do something that helps you remember who you are as an individual.

Socialization is as important as exercise or relaxation but is often the last requirement considered. It takes a special effort to avoid the isolation that dementia and its caregiving imposes. However, there is a growing pool of research shows that socialization is as important as exercise in lowering the risk of dementia.[22] It also helps to decrease dementia symptoms in Persons already living with dementia. Humans are social creatures who need social contact to function well.

I make it a point to add social interactions to our lives. I have a standing date to go to lunch with a friend once a week while Larry is in daycare. We go to church too. I choose the early service; it's smaller and easier for Larry to deal with. And then there are the grandkids. My daughter brings them over here. Larry always loves that. Well, I do too. And it is much easier to have them here where Larry can escape to his room if things get too busy for him. -- Doris

As interests narrow to what's happening with your Person, it is easy to forget to be responsive to your own needs; to avoid returning calls from friends, and eventually never see or talk with them at all. A good way to start being social is to attend a support group. Group members find they have much in common and it makes it easier to stay in contact.

Putting it all together. You may have noticed that many of these basic needs overlap. For example, every one of the needs mentioned, from getting enough sleep to being social can act to decrease stress. The physical needs, such as sleep, hydration and nutrition all work together to give you better health, which may allow you to require less medical care. Spirituality is an entity of its own, but care partners often practice it in ways that are very social and you will likely want to use some of your personal time for maintenance. We don't have only physical, psychological, spiritual or social needs. We, as humans, need them all!

***

Responsive Care Takeaways for Basic Needs:

- A care partner is the Person's most valuable dementia care tool.

  Attitude: Recognize your value.

  Action: Take good care of yourself.

- Care partners are prone to long-term stress with temporary dementia-like symptoms.

  Action: Recognize your limitations and get the help you need.

- People need 7-9 hours of sleep a night.

  Action: If the Person's sleep habits cause too much sleep disruption, a spouse may need to sleep in a separate bed or bedroom.

- People need about 8 glasses of fluid per day.

  Actions:

  o Add regular times to drink water to your daily routine.

  o Monitor your urine color to be sure you are drinking enough fluid.

- The Mediterranean diet provides good nutrition.

  Action: Substitute fruit, or a pleasurable activity for starchy comfort food.

- Exercising fights stress and improves health.

  Action: Find a way to exercise that works for you and make it a part of your routine.

- Medical care is as important for the care partner as for the Person.

  Action: Make and keep regular appointments and follow the doctor's orders.

- Spirituality provides an inner strength and a sense of purpose that decreases depression and anxiety.

  Action: Develop your faith and use it regularly.

- Personal time is a must for emotional health.

  Action: Find a way to fit something that helps you remember who you are into your own schedule on a regular basis.

- Socialization is as important for the care partner as it is for Person.

  Action: Take the time to answer calls, go to lunch with a friend and maintain organizational memberships.

11. Caregiving Is Not a One-Person Job

overextension: *Doing more than one can do and still have time and energy for self-care.*

burnout: *physical, emotional and mental exhaustion so great that it is difficult to be positive and caring.*

compassion fatigue: *Extreme state of stress resulting in feelings of hopelessness, indifference, pessimism and lack of empathy.*

***

Caregiver burnout is common in any caregiver situation, more common with dementia and even more common when the dementia is LBD. It starts with overextension and sneaks up on you gradually. You start out as a partnership, with the Person able to do most of what they've always done. As their abilities decrease and their needs increase, you take on more and more of the load. You may not notice the changes until you realize that your own needs aren't getting met--or more likely, someone else notices and calls it to your attention. If you ignore this heads-up, your next step is burnout.

I can't remember worth beans; I'm irritable all the time and I have no patience. I'm making stupid mistakes. Yesterday, I almost dropped Nathan because I forgot how to transfer him. -- Elsie

Elsie is experiencing burnout symptoms--fuzzy cognition, irritability, impatience, and fatigue. Yes, stress symptoms--stress carried to extremes! She really isn't safe anymore, not for Nathan or for herself. If she doesn't get help soon, something is likely to happen: an injury, an illness, or even death--more likely hers than Nathan's.

I'm so tired. I just don't care anymore. I want to and I feel guilty that I can't, but I just don't. I actually find myself hiding out in the bathroom to avoid Nathan. -- Elsie

Elsie is also experiencing compassion fatigue, an extreme form of burnout where empathy is lost. This is even more serious than burnout because she has lost the ability to care.

Warning signs of compassion fatigue include all of those related to burnout plus feeling overwhelmed, exhausted and drained, avoiding your loved one, loss of patience and tolerance, increased anxiety and difficulty making care decisions.

Any care partner will experience the above symptoms occasionally. Use them as a warning to re-evaluate your life. Do what you must to add back into your life some of the basic needs talked about in Chapter 11.

I recognized that I was getting so involved in caregiving that I had let all of my other interests go. Some days are awful and I feel like I just don't want to go on. I used to love to garden, but I don't get outside much anymore now that Carol takes most of my attention. I used to enjoy reading but I don't seem to have time for that either. -- Harold

Harold is beginning to experience bouts of compassion fatigue. It isn't a regular thing yet and he can still make changes that will improve his life, and by extension, Carol's. He has made the first step. He recognizes the problem, which can sometimes be the most important step. Next he needs to decrease his stress by adding some of those basic needs back into his life. If he doesn't take these steps, the stress will get worse and he will be facing a crisis.

When the definition for compassion fatigue describes your daily life rather than a bad day, you need help. This is as serious as a physical problem such as a broken leg or a damaged back. You should not be acting as a caregiver in this condition. For your safety and the Person's, you must find respite care until you are again able to take on the job.

Getting help means not only help with caregiving but also help dealing with your own issues. Once you have reduced your stress level enough to think clearly and feel empathetically, you will be able to make some decisions that will help you to continue as a care partner while taking care of yourself as well. Care facilities are very aware of burnout and compassion fatigue and they set up policies to prevent it. Home care partners have to be their own advocates. You have to identify and set your own limits. This is seldom easy to do.

Care partners often say, "I know I should take better care of myself but I just can't because...."

I don't have the time. The usual cry we hear when we talk about self-care is: "...how can I do everything I need to do for my loved one and still have time for me?"

This response signals that it is time for more help. Care partners in a recent poll[23] reported that what they regretted most was not getting help soon enough. Of course being responsive to your need for help isn't enough. You need to make it happen. If you are unsure of how to do this, talk to other support group members or to the Area Agency on Aging in your community.

I promised. Promises can stop you from getting help. The second most common mistakes caregivers make, according to the above poll, is telling their loved one that they would never place them in a residential facility.

I promised Annie I would always keep her at home. When I was unable to do this, she became very angry and never forgave me. She couldn't understand that I had no choice-- that keeping her at home was no longer safe. -- James

Be responsive to your Person's inability to understand extenuating circumstances. While it is very understandable that a Person will wish to stay home in familiar territory, this is often not possible for the whole journey. Furthermore, it is likely to be your health, rather than theirs, that gives out first. This will not be something the Person will be able to understand. Better to promise something like, "*I'll do everything I can to keep you safe and comfortable.*"

We can't afford it. Another very valid concern concerns a lack of funds to pay for help.

We've always been frugal. Tony and I have always done our own repairs and even did most of the work when we added an extra bedroom to our house. We have limited resources and I hate to think of wasting them for something that I've always done, always been able to do. Our daughter comes over and helps out occasionally but she has her own family responsibilities and so she can't do much. -- Angela

Dementia care is expensive. Much of it is probably work that you have been doing for years. That can make it hard to justify the cost of additional help. Like Angela, many care partners keep struggling along, saying that they can do it, long after they need help.

Re-evaluate if you hear yourself say "I'd like more help but we can't afford it for things I've always done. I'll manage somehow." Notice how much more demanding and time

112

consuming your caregiving tasks have become. This is no longer only the work you've always done!

Caregiver illness and even death is a very real danger. Far more dementia caregivers become ill or die than do similar people in the general population, or even other caregivers.[24] The stress, and therefore the risk, is even greater with dementia.

If you become so ill that you can't function--or worse, if you die, the cost will be even greater. That doesn't even take into account what your own healthcare costs will be. The Person will still need the help but you won't be able to fill in the gaps or provide the necessary emotional support.

There are ways to obtain help even if your finances are tight. The Area Agency on Aging and other members in your support group can help you find the state, military and other agencies that offer financial help. Count on there being waiting periods and other requirements, but the funds are often there if you search for them.

Transportation is just too difficult. Having difficulty with transfers and transportation may be the signal to a care partner that help is needed.

We used to go out for a drive but the whole process of getting Leon in and out of a car has become a nightmare. It's too scary to do unless we really have to. I'm afraid he will fall or I'll hurt my back. -- Carla

Optional outings that used to be enjoyable fall by the wayside with both Person and care partner becoming more isolated.

Such difficulties are a warning that it is time to consider getting regular help. In the meantime, most communities have a service such as Dial-a-Ride. You can make an appointment for a strong, qualified driver to come to your home, help you load the Person and their wheelchair into their van, take the two of you to your destination and bring you home later. The cost for these services is usually minimal. The Eldercare Locator offers a pamphlet on transportation options for seniors.[25] Contact your Agency on Aging or Senior Center for local information.

My way is best. Care partners often say, "Others can't give the care that I do."

I hate to think of putting Bob in a residential facility. I know he won't get the kind of care I give him. I know just what he likes and doesn't, the best way to get him to do things, and just what pleases him most...or sets him off for that matter. At home he is the only one but there he'd be one of many. Who knows how long he'd have to wait for help when he needs it? -- Joy

Joy's right. They probably won't give Bob the kind of personalized care that she does. But how long is she going to be able to do so--and do it effectively, without experiencing those telltale dementia symptoms herself?

Actually, Joy won't give up the most important part of her job when Bob enters a facility. Her job changes, but it is every bit as important. The staff does the tiring physical stuff while Joy continues to provide a lot of responsive care: critical emotional and social support. She also has information that only she knows. She can provide information about Bob's routines, likes and dislikes. This will keep Bob comfortable and make the staff's job easier.

Caregiver Questionnaire. The Caregiver Questionnaire in the Resources Section of this book (Appendix B) provides questions to ask yourself to see where you are in this process. Get a head start by regularly reviewing these questions. If you find that it is time for you to seek help, don't put it off. In fact, start your research right away so that when you do need help you can get it sooner.

Also check out the National Caregiver's Library[26]. It has a huge list of resources for care partners.

Making the changes necessary to take care of yourself don't have to happen all at once. If you catch yourself before you've slipped all the way into compassion fatigue you can start small and gradually build a routine that will keep both of you safer, happier and healthier. Take just five minutes to do something for yourself, read a book, dance, talk to a friend, go for a walk. Then gradually expand that.

***

Responsive Care Takeaways for Caregiving is not a One Person Job:

- Overextending is a gradual thing; others may notice that you need help before you do.

  Action: Do regular reviews of your needs.

- Caregiver burnout symptoms include fuzzy and negative thinking, fatigue, depression, illnesses, irritability and isolation.

- Burnout is a safety issue. An overly-stressed care partner is not safe to care for the Person or themselves.

  Action: It is time to get help when you notice you are experiencing "dementia" symptoms or don't have time and energy left for your own self-care.

- Compassion fatigue is caregiver burnout that has advanced to include the inability to feel empathy.

  Action: View even an occasional day of this as a danger signal and institute changes in your life that will decrease stress before it gets worse.

- Ongoing compassion fatigue is an emergency situation as serious as a care partner's debilitating injury would be.

  Action: Any care partner who finds themselves experiencing compassion fatigue on a daily basis needs to get respite care and seek help immediately.

- Feeling that you don't have time for self-care is a sign that you need help with caregiving tasks.

  Action: Prioritize your self-care needs and see them as important as those tasks related more directly to caregiving.

- Promises like "I'll never put you in a residential center" can backfire when your health gives out.

  Action: Be careful what you promise.

- Paying for help is not as expensive as paying for injuries and illnesses caused by burnout or compassion fatigue.

  Action: Ask family for help, research community resources and pay for help if still needed.

- Caregiving can become so physically difficult that the Person or care partner is in danger of physical injury.

  Action: Accept that it is time for help and do it.

- Most communities have resources for physical and financial help.

  Action: Research these resources and use them.

12. Become an Improv Actor

communication: An interaction where words and actions are based on the same reality.

therapeutic fibbing: *Speaking from the Person's reality rather than your own in order to avoid increased anxiety and agitation.*

improvisational (improv) theater: *a form of live theater where the dialogue, story and characters are created by the actors as the action unfolds in present time.*

improv acting: *Putting one's own reality on hold--leaving it off the stage--and playing your given part with conviction in the Person's drama.*

***

"What?" you say. "With all I have to do, now you want me to take up acting?"

Yes, learning to be an improv actor can reduce stress and improve communication.

Nathan and I have always agreed not to lie to each other. My support group has talked about "therapeutic fibbing," and going along with what he says. To me, that sounds too much like lying. I don't want to start that now, especially not about something so offensive as being unfaithful. I'd never do that! - Elsie

The problem is that Nathan can only see a reality where Elsie has already been unfaithful and is now lying about it. Because Nathan is stuck with this, so is Elsie. She knows that Nathan experiences her "honest" defending and explaining as so much more betrayal. Even so, the idea of therapeutic fibbing just feels wrong.

Elsie isn't alone. It isn't that therapeutic fibbing doesn't work. It does. Used appropriately, it meets the criteria for working with delusions: It involves recognizing the Person's different world-view (reality) and responding with words (little white lies) that soothe but don't harm.

However many people, care partners and professionals alike, react negatively to the idea of lying to the Person. Care partners like Elsie say that lying has never been a part of their relationship and they aren't going to start now. Professionals warn that you can get caught in the lies, causing distrust and even more agitation.

Improv avoids the "lying vs. truth" controversy, while helping Elsie enter Nathan's world-view, where communication is possible. It works with, instead of against, the Person while allowing the care partner to maintain their own sense of reality.

It's easier to go along with Nathan when I think of myself as an improv actor. I'm not lying; I'm playing a role in Nathan's drama. It's like when I was a little girl and Daddy drank my imaginary tea. He didn't feel he had to tell me the cup was empty. He just played the part I gave him and "drank" the tea. Now I'm the one playing the part. – Elsie

When Elsie views the interaction as a drama where Nathan sets the stage, it is much easier for her to put her own reality on hold and step into Nathan's reality, where communication is possible. Like a good actor, she doesn't have to believe his drama; she just has to play her part convincingly.

It is important that Elsie be sincere. Persons living with dementia are experts at sensing phoniness. That's one reason why seeing herself as an actor is better than simply lying. She can think of how she'd really feel in this situation and act it out.

Improv is like real life in that there is no plot and the conversation is made up as the players go along. The common concept of improv acting is that it is a form of comedy, but this does not have to be. It can be about any situation at all.

An improv actor does not get to choose the script, but they do choose how to react. Likewise, a care partner doesn't get to choose what the Person presents to them, *but they can choose how to respond.* And that is the magic! By choosing effective ways of responding, the care partner can allow the Person to feel understood, valued--and soothed.

Annie: Look! There are children coming into the living room from behind the TV. (Sounds agitated)

James: (looks behind the TV) Hmm. I don't see a door, but hey kids, it's time to go home. Out this way, (Ushers them out the front door.) Bye now. (Closes the door.)

Listen. Truly listen to what the Person has to say. Listen without judgment, without planning how to answer. Listen especially for the emotions involved. These are often more important than the words. James recognized Annie's agitation and knew the kids were bothering her.

Agree. An improv actor accepts what's offered and goes with it. Agree in action if not in words. James let his actions show that he accepted Annie's reality by going to look for a door behind the TV. *Agreeing is not the same as believing.* Agreeing is simply recognizing that you hear the Person and will act out your part in the drama.

Contribute. Add something non-conflicting that moves the action on. Here's where you have some control. You can choose the direction you want the action to go. James moved the action in the direction he thought would be most helpful when he ushered the "kids" out the door. Because his choice didn't conflict with Annie's reality, she easily accepted it and relaxed.

Accept change. Perhaps one of the most important parts of improv acting is the willingness to go with the flow, to respond to change quickly and move on. This is also true for dementia caregiving. Dementia is progressive and will continually change both the Person and the care involved. Demanding that things stay the same only brings stress and frustration.

It used to be that I could tell Annie that the things she saw weren't real but now that just upsets her and so I don't argue with her. -- James

When James accepted that Annie's view of her hallucinations had changed, he stopped trying to explain them away and went with the flow.

Accept the Person's reality. Accepting change also includes accepting the Person's new reality--without judgment. Their version is the only one that counts, the only one where effective communication is possible. Avoid explaining, defending or arguing for YOUR reality.

Here's what happened when Elsie uses improv with Nathan's accusations of infidelity:

Nathan (angry voice): I know you went to see your boyfriend instead of going to the store.

Elsie: (calm, sincere voice): I'm sorry. (Takes responsibility for Nathan's anger. Accepts that this is Nathan's scene, where he has cast her as the bad guy.) You must have been really worried. (Speaks to his fears, not his anger.)

Nathan (calmer, but still hanging onto his anger): I was. I know you are making plans to run off with him.

Elsie: I'm sorry. (As long as there is anger, Elsie soothes it with apologies.) That must be scary to think about. (Continues to focus on the fear, not the anger.)

Nathan: Of course it's scary. But I know that you will leave. I know you are tired of caring for me.

Elsie: I'm sorry. I do get tired sometimes. (Responds to the part of his complaint that she can agree with.) You do too, don't you. (Changes the subject and includes Nathan.)

Nathan: (sighs) Yes, I do. (Calmer now.)

Elsie: Remember when we had all the energy in the world? (Moves the action further away from Nathan's accusation.) Remember the fun times we had, like when we went to the beach? I loved spending a whole week there with you. (Smiles and takes Nathan's hand.)

Nathan (smiles back): Yes, that was fun. (Pats her hand.)

Elsie: Oh, and I brought you a snack. I know you love these. (Digs in her grocery bag and hands Nathan a small bag of chips— a bribe, more distraction.)

Nathan had set the scene in this drama and cast Elsie in her role as the bad guy. Like a good improv actor, she accepted the role, responded to Nathan's feelings and then moved the action into a more pleasant direction, with more comfortable positive feelings.

Be in the moment. Improv is all about what is happening this minute--and the feelings involved right now. So is dementia. The Person lives in the here and now. When Nathan accused

Elsie of infidelity, all that mattered was that moment when Nathan's fear of abandonment showed up in his delusions. It didn't matter that they'd been married for fifty years and she had never been unfaithful. That's in the past. Nathan could only deal with right now. When Elsie entered Nathan's reality, he was able to accept her apology let go of some of his anger.

Focus on the emotion. Good acting involves responding in a believable way to the emotions of others. As dementia progresses one's thinking is often replaced with emotion. Improv allowed Elsie to ignore Nathan's verbal accusation and focus on his feelings. She apologized to defuse his anger—she truly was sorry for his pain. Then, as a friend and not an enemy, she was able to use reminiscing to move the action towards more positive feelings. Elsie's mention of the beach brought up residual positive feelings that she used to help override his negative ones. If, like Elsie, you pay less attention to accusations and more to the underlying feelings, you will be more successful.

Accept offers and gifts. When an improv actor is offered an imaginary gift, the actor takes it and runs with it, adding information and action. Take what the Person offers, be it a hallucination, a memory (real or false) or a comment (pleasing or not) and find some value in it. Show appreciation, talk about feelings, and ask for more information.

Larry: When I got my engineering degree, I was so excited. I got top grades in my class.

Doris: Oh, that is impressive. You must be very proud of that. (Doris waits for Larry to say more.)

Doris knows that Larry never went to college, but she accepts his "gift" of information and shows interest with her question. Be careful with questions. Make them too difficult and the Person will become frustrated. You don't want those negative emotions! Sometimes, simply showing interest and waiting, as Doris did, is enough. Then the Person can volunteer more as they like.

Develop options. Persons living with dementia respond with knee-jerk actions because their brains don't give them a choice. Responsive care involves considering responses and choosing the best one. Like improv actors, you can reject "I don't like what just happened," and instead ask, "What can I do with what just happened? How can I make it work for us?" This takes knowing what doesn't work as well as what does.

Carol: I want to go home. I don't like it here.

Harold: (nod) You want to go home.

Carol: Yes, I don't like it here.

Harold: Can you tell me what you don't like?

Carol: (fidgeting) Uh, I don't know. I just don't like it here.

Harold (to self: oh, oh, too hard a question.) Well, does your tummy hurt? (She has a history of this, so it is a good guess.)

Carol: Yes. I want to go home where I feel better.

Harold: Yes, being home does feel good. Would you like to take some antacid lozenges to see if that helps you feel better?

Carol: (considers it) Then will you take me home?

Harold: Of course, but for now, here's an antacid lozenge, OK?

Harold rejected explaining, defending and arguing as ineffective. Instead, he repeated Carol's request as a statement, showing he understood. Then he moved the action forward, by asking specific questions about how she felt, based on his knowledge of her issues. When he realized that his question was too difficult, he rephrased it to be more specific. He moved away from Carol's negative feelings by offering help and a promise. *Warning: Be careful about promises that you can't either keep or deflect.*

Use small steps and invitations, not force. Improv actors sometimes start out with an agenda, but they have to work to make it acceptable to their audience. Caregivers often have an agenda too. For example, Harold's agenda was to help Carol feel more at home.

Carol (after she's taken the antacid lozenges): I want to go home. This isn't home.

Harold: (nods) You want to go home. Would you like to rest a little first? That always makes you feel better.

Carol: OK, then can we go home?

Small steps and suggestions that are more of an invitation make an agenda more acceptable. Harold's first step was the antacid lozenges, his second was the nap. Carol is likely to wake up from her nap feeling at home. If she doesn't, Harold's next step might be to take her for an enjoyable ride and bring her "home."

Commit 100%. Improv actors have to be willing to commit to BEING their character. In that moment, they ARE whoever they portray and they speak as their character would speak. Caregivers must do this too. When you accept a role in the Person's drama, you must play the part with conviction. For example, when Nathan accused Elsie of infidelity, she was not only sorry that he was hurt. She went further and thought about how she'd feel if his accusation was true and knew

124

she'd really want be forgiven. With this in mind, she was able to speak with conviction, making it easier for Nathan to believe her and let go of his painful negative feelings.

Use touch. Gentle touch is powerful. You don't always need words to set a scene or move it forward. You probably touch your loved one a lot, just getting work done. You touch while helping with dressing, bedtime, and bathroom duties, eating, sitting, etc. That's not the same as meaningful touching, like hugging, holding hands or a pat on the back as your pass. These touches show you care, that you really want to be in this relationship.

(*Warning:* When a Person is behaving in a way that could become violent, DO NOT get within touching distance until they have calmed down.) Elsie didn't touch Nathan while he was angry and accusing her of infidelity. But once he calmed down, she took his hand and held it, showing him nonverbally that she cared and wanted to be with him.

Collaborate. Improv acting is not done alone. For a skit to move forward, the actors must work together. Imagine what it would be like if you went to a comedy club and heard these two improv actors:

Paul: Hi, Amy. Want to come on a ride through the forest?

Amy: Sure, I'll drive us around the city. Here' a shopping center. (Doesn't accept Paul's drama but offers one of her own.)

Paul: I see a forest trail. (Still inviting Amy into his drama.)

Amy: There are high-rises here and lots of people. (Ignores Paul.)

Paul (showing anger): Look, there are some deer and a creek. Why don't you see them?

Amy (patiently): They aren't there, Paul. I only see city streets.

Paul, (stomping his foot): There are no streets here. Only trees.

Unless either Amy or Paul accepts the other's drama, their skit will fail; it has nowhere to go. Amy's patient and insistent efforts didn't work. They just made Paul angry. Here either actor could give in and accept the other's view. Paul could go to the city or Amy could drive in the forest.

Caregiving is a little different. Just as with improv, the action moves forward only if the two of you work together towards a common goal. The Person's is stuck with what their damaged brain chooses. But you can choose to stay in your own reality or to accept the Person's. If, as with Elsie, this puts you in the "bad guy" role, so be it. When Elsie didn't work with Nathan, he perceived her as a lying opponent. When she entered Nathan's drama, she was no longer the enemy and could work with him to move towards a less painful direction.

Improv actors collaborate with people off the stage as well. They solicit help from the audience, from people not directly involved in the action. "Give us a task, a place, an idea to pursue," they ask. Care partners need to reach out and ask for help too. I know you've heard this before. But are you still trying to do it all? Get someone to help a few hours a week at least. *Caregiving is not a one-person job.*

Improv actors also collaborate together, sharing ideas, feedback and friendship. Likewise, care partners need to surround themselves with others in similar situations. Caregiving can be isolating. You must make an effort to find others with whom you can relate, share ideas, resources, laughter and tears. Join a caregiver support group. Have a "phone buddy," someone you can vent with, laugh with and just be relaxed with.

Give yourself permission to fail. It is human nature to want to do the best you can. But trying to be the "perfect caregiver" comes with too much stress, a set up for failure in itself.

When improv actors make mistakes, they shrug or laugh and try something else. Researchers are more serious about failure. They view it as an important part of the discovery process, a ruling out of what doesn't work so that they can figure out what does. You can do both. Like a researcher, you can accept failure as a valuable learning experience. Then, like an improv actor, you can forgive yourself and move on.

***

Responsive Care Takeaways for Become an Improv Actor:

- Improv acting allows a care partner to enter a Person's reality in a way that feels less like deceitful.
- You must play the script the Person chooses; but you can choose how to play it out.

Attitudes:

  o An acceptance that that you can change but they can't.
  o A 100% commitment to being believable.
  o A positive, constructive attitude rather than a negative response to a hurtful statement.
  o A forgiving, constructive attitude about failure.

Actions:

- o Listen with an open mind, being alert for emotions.
- o Use verbal or nonverbal agreement to show that you accept your role in the Person's drama.
- o Contribute something that will move the action in the direction you want it to go without conflict.
- o Stay in the moment, and in the here and now.
- o Respond to the Person's underlying emotions and ignore the irrational words.
- o Accept gifts such as stories and avoid discounting them.
- o Continue to move the action forward in small steps.
- o Use invitations, not directives.
- o Use touch to express caring. (but not if the Person is angry and possibly dangerous.)
- o Collaborate with other care partners, sharing ideas and friendship.

13. Being Flexible

flexibility: *The ability to cope with changes and think about tasks in creative ways.*

inflexibility: *Rigid and stuck on one's old ways, often caused by immobilizing negative emotions like fear and worry.*

guilt: *An emotion triggered by perceived wrongdoing that becomes destructive when used as a method for trying to control the past.*

worry: *An emotion triggered by concern about a future event that becomes destructive when used to try to control that event.*

***

Because their job is so important, care partners often have higher expectations for themselves than for others. Wallowing in guilt and self-blame, they believe that if they lose patience, or don't do something as it "should be done," then they have failed.

Improv actors practice flexibility. When jokes go flat or scenes don't make sense, they take it all in stride. Their failures don't define them as people or as actors. They laugh, let it go and move on. "Well, that didn't work. How else can I do that, so that it will work next time?

Being flexible helps you let go of unrealistic expectations and stop being stuck by using failure as a badge of shame. Instead, see failure as a part of the process. See it as a learning tool, reminder or warning, as one more step toward your goal.

Being flexible is a process:

- Recognizing the problem or the failure
- Looking for the lesson
- Experiencing any guilt involved and making amends
- Worrying a little and looking for a better way
- Taking action
- Trying again and again
- Moving on

Let's break each of these down:

Recognize the problem. Sometimes that's easy. The Person expresses discomfort with a behavior such as yelling. Often, it's less clear.

Last night, Steve watched a detective story on TV. Then I think he chased those bad guys all night long in his dreams. -- Rhonda

It only took Rhonda a sleepless night for her to see that it had been a mistake to let Steve watch such an exciting show. When the care partner has the problem, such as feeling overwhelmed, it can sometimes take something as serious as a fall.

Feel the guilt and look for the lesson. Guilt's job is to trigger you into expressing your concern to anyone you may have hurt (including yourself!) and to point out the need to try a different way. Then, guilt's job is over.

He's been watching that show for years. I guess it is too exciting for him now. I should have noticed this sooner. -- Rhonda

Forgive yourself. The next step is to forgive. Be as gentle and compassionate with yourself as you are with others. Making even a serious mistake does not make you a bad care partner. You aren't perfect. You don't have to be! Love yourself anyway. This self-caring will be mirrored by the Person as positive feelings.

I guess I'm not perfect! Oh, well. -- Rhonda

It was natural for Rhonda to feel guilty, but she didn't cling to it. She let it go when its work was done.

Worry a little and look for a better way. A moderate amount of worry can lead to constructive evaluations and motivate you to take action. What can I do? Who should I ask? What are my options? What else can I try? Can I think of anything better?

I remembered that someone in my support group talked about using DVDs with old TV programs and I decided to give that a try. – Rhonda

Rhonda worried enough to gather some information, and then she let the worry go. Its job was done.

Take action. This might mean that you'll set up a plan of what to do later. Or it may mean that you'll do something right away.

I ordered some old programs for Steve to watch instead of his detective stories. -- Rhonda

There needs to be a feeling of "doing" involved, as when Rhonda ordered the DVDs, to help you let go of the guilt and worry and move on. The doing doesn't have to be action. It might be the decision to do nothing.

Try, try again. If the first thing you try doesn't work, try again. Being willing to try something different is a big part of being flexible.

The first one I tried had too much action in it and made him restless at night. Then I tried another and he hated it--"too mushy," he told me. Finally, I put in The Andy Griffin Show. He likes it and it doesn't make him restless. -- Rhonda

Being flexible often means trying more than one thing. If one doesn't work, what else might? Try that. Rhonda tried several programs before she found one that worked for Steve.

Let go of negative emotions and move on. Once guilt and worry have done their job, it is time to let them go. All too often people hang onto these and try to use them to control the past and future. "If I can't do anything else, at least I can feel guilty or worry about it." The truth is that these are both negative emotions and they will not only make Rhonda feel worse, they will be reflected by Steve as unwanted behaviors.

We are both happy campers! – Rhonda

Rhonda is focusing on her success, not the failures that led up to it.

Lighten up. Add some humor to the situation. If you can laugh about a negative experience, it won't feel nearly as devastating.

I told my support group about our adventures with the DVDs and we all had a good laugh. I'd still been carrying around some bad feelings about that, thinking I should have been able to choose better right away. But after laughing about it, I feel so much better. -- Rhonda

Laughing with the group helped Rhonda to see that she was still carrying around unreasonable expectations about her actions and to let them go.

Flexibility may mean lowering your standards. Your house doesn't have to be spick and span. The dishes can pile up for a day or more. The Person doesn't have to have a clean change of clothes every day, etc.

It was such a job to convince Steve to take a shower that I just quit doing it every day. He was happier and I was less burdened. – Rhonda

Being flexible allowed Rhonda to give up a certain amount of cleanliness to have less conflict and cut down on her workload.

Flexibility comes into effect with finances too. Dementia care is expensive. Even with help from the state or other sources, you may not be able to afford what you really want. Don't let this stop you from getting the best help you *can* afford.

I knew that Steve needed 24/7 care but our finances were limited. We got help from the state and I finally found a wonderful assisted care facility. I wanted Steve to have his own room but our finances wouldn't stretch to cover the difference between what the state paid and the extra cost for a private room. -- Rhonda

Like Rhonda and Steve, you can seldom have it all. You just have to make the best choice you can with the resources you have, let go of what might have been, and move on.

Steve and his roommate squabbled a lot. I took Steve out of the room to other parts of the building when I was there and that helped. -- Rhonda

Moving on doesn't necessarily mean accepting a difficult situation without trying to change it. It is important to identify what needs to change. Rhonda didn't try to stop Steve and his roommate from squabbling. That would have been futile, since both had dementia. Instead, she separated the roommates.

I talked to the staff about the squabbling. They were concerned too. They changed Steve to a different room with a more compatible roommate. He is so much happier now. -- Rhonda

Part of being flexible involves recognizing when you need help -- and asking for it. Rhonda sought help from an outside source with more power than she had to change the situation. Again, Rhonda changed Steve's environment; she didn't try to change him.

Look for the fun. Being flexible means loosening up. Caregiving is definitely one of the most important jobs a care partner will ever have. The Person is often totally dependent on how you do your job. It can feel like an overwhelming responsibility. Yes, it can get scary. Then add to that the fact that the Person is probably scared as well. This is a new country for them too.

All of the above is true. But it also true that you can find humor in almost anything if you just look for it. Humor is a healthy way to lighten all those heavy feelings of responsibility, of always needing to be perfect, of feeling like a failure. Just laugh. It takes flexibility to do this, to move from the seriousness of your task to a little bit of light-heartedness, but the rewards are huge. It helps you to see things more positively, which can go a long way towards reducing your fear and theirs. Look for the fun, the jokes, the chances to laugh and the many reasons to smile. Humor can make any job easier. Use it often.

***

Responsive Care Takeaways for Being Flexible:

- Being flexible is about letting go of unreasonable expectations, forgiving your mistakes, learning from them and moving on with a positive attitude.
- Being flexible is a process:
  - Own the problem or failure as part of a process.
  - Find for the lesson.
  - Let guilt drive you to make amends.
  - Let worry drive you to look for a better way.
  - Use humor to help you see the positives.
  - Take action.
  - Try again and again.
  - Move on.
- Guilt and worry are useful but when their job is done, they become destructive.

Attitudes:

  - A positive, can-do attitude makes it easier to be flexible.
  - Use humor to smooth the way for both of you.
  - Lowered standards that allow you to cut down on workload and meet financial responsibilities.
  - Accept that you can't do it all and that you WILL need help at times .
  - Be willing to adapt and try a different way.

Actions:

- o Recognize the problem or failure as part of a process, not the end result. Look for what you can change.
- o Look for the lesson--not the blame.
- o Let yourself feel any guilt that come. Did you hurt anyone, including yourself?
- o Make amends and forgive yourself. Then let the guilt go; it's done its job.
- o Worry a little and look for a better way. Then let go of the worry and take action.
- o Did that work? If not, try again. Repeat the process as many times as you need to.
- o Move on with a positive attitude. Leave guilt and worry behind.
- o Add humor to make everything a little easier.

14. Being Positive

reacting: *Making an immediate, usually negative, response to a situation.*

responding: *Making a more thought-out response to a situation.*

making a conscious choice: *Taking the time to use abstract thinking to evaluate a situation and decide upon a response.*

***

The more positive you are, the happier and healthier you will be. Positive people have less risk for most diseases, including dementia, depression, heart disease and even the common cold. Especially important for the care partner, being positive also lowers stress and helps you cope better with issues such as dementia-related behaviors.

As a care partner, you are actually being positive for two. Although a positive attitude is equally helpful for the Person, they have less ability to make those conscious choices necessary to stay positive. They will react to whatever emotion is strongest and most persistent--often something negative, and therefore stronger than the gentler positive emotions. For example, they don't have delusions about how you happily found their lost slippers or that you came back from the store with a gift for them. No they have delusions about what they fear--that their slippers are irrevocably lost or that you are planning to leave and won't be coming back at all.

Gordon tends to see the negatives first but I've noticed that if I stay positive, it is a lot easier for him to be positive too. Once in a while I catch myself following his lead and we both get to be negative for a while. Thank goodness, I've learned

how to catch myself and change to a more positive outlook! --
Virginia

Emotions are contagious. As Virginia found, she could easily get caught in Gordon's negativity. However, she can model being positive and Gordon will follow suit and be much more positive than he could by himself. Thus, modeling a positive world view helps the Person to be happier and more content with fewer behaviors.

This isn't always easy. It is not only the Person who pays attention first to those strong negative emotions. We all do. As nature's alarm system, they demand attention and action. However, just as you would with a smoke alarm that goes off when you burn the toast, you can make a conscious choice to turn this alarm off and choose a more positive view of the event.

Making a conscious choice involves abstract thinking and this takes time. Often one's reaction to an event is immediate, with little or no consideration of how to view the event or respond to it. Given that negative emotions are stronger, such an automatic reaction will more than likely be negative. In addition, humans are creatures of habit. Once they've reacted in a certain way to an event, they will likely react that way again and again--unless they make a conscious choice to change.

Making the change. You may be more negative than you'd like to be but you can change. While it is true that you are designed to pay careful attention to the negatives, you are also given the capability to enjoy the positives.

I used to think "Oh, that's going to be hard. I don't know if we will be able to do that. Now I think, "That will be a challenge but I'm sure we'll figure out how to do it. -- Virginia

Virginia didn't get from thinking negatively to thinking positively overnight. Here's some steps to get you started, along with Virginia's comments about her experiences:

- **Be aware.** Notice how much you focus on the negatives. You must help a Person let go of stronger negative thinking before you can move them on. It is the same for you. You must become aware of the negatives and consciously let them go before you can move on to being positive.

I was surprised at how many times my thoughts were negative. I had thought I was basically positive until I started being more aware of my thoughts. -- Virginia

- **Cultivate positive friends.** Positivity and negativity are both contagious. Choosing to spend time with friends and family who have positive attitudes will make it much easier for you to choose to be positive.

I don't get out much but I do spend some time on the internet. I've begun choosing to ignore posts by people who are negative and focus on those that are more positive. I've noticed that my posts have become a lot more positive too. -- Virginia

- **Make small changes.** Choose just one type of negative thinking to change at a time. If you try to change your whole attitude all at once, you will be much more likely to give up in frustration.

The first thing I worked on was what made me the most frustrated. Gordon gets up several times a night and by the last one, I'm a real witch, because I'm not getting enough sleep. I worked on being more pleasant to him, but I also stopped blaming myself for being cranky when I was tired. I was actually surprised to notice that Gordon wasn't as restless when I was better natured. He even got up less! Wow! -- Virginia

- *Take time.* Don't react immediately. Give yourself some time to think it through, consider how you might respond and to choose a more positive response. The few seconds this takes will make the difference between an immediate reaction and a thought-out response.

Now before I act, I take what I call a "thought break." Just this has made me more positive because I don't automatically choose a negative reaction. -- Virginia

- *Make it a habit.* As you repeat these steps over and over, your conscious choices will become habit and take so little time it will seem as though you aren't even thinking about it anymore. But you are. You are still choosing to be positive over being negative. It has simply become "second nature."

It took me a long time to automatically smile and be pleasant with Gordon when he got up for the third time. But it isn't as hard anymore. I guess it has become enough of a habit that I can do it even when I'm tired. -- Virginia

- *Be patient.* It used to be thought that creating a new habit took three weeks. It can actually take a couple of months or longer.

Staying Positive

There are many things you can do that will make you more positive and help the Person to be more positive as well.

- *Treat yourself as a friend.* Instead of negative self-talk about something that didn't go right, tell yourself the same thing you might say to a friend. Reword your self-talk to be encouraging rather than derogatory.

This idea really made an impression on me. I realized that I'd never tell a friend how stupid they were or that they had made a horrible mess of their project. I wouldn't even tell an enemy the sort of things I used to say to myself. Now I try to say the same things to myself that I'd say to a friend. -- Virginia

Those negative thoughts can stay with you for a long time. Let them go and give yourself some positive encouragement instead.

A nurse told me once that for every put-down there must be five push-ups. I think about that now and if I do notice that I've been tough on myself, I try to think of five good things about me. Sometimes I can't think of any except that I'm still trying, but it all helps. -- Virginia

Virginia is right. It takes a lot of positive thoughts to negate just one negative one. However, making that conscious choice to see yourself positively is definitely worth the effort.

- *Give a gift.* Gifting helps both you and the person who receives your gift. It doesn't have to be material. Caregiving can become more job than "loving help" but an extra pat or hug becomes a gift. Giving a gift triggers your own feel-good hormones once when you choose it, once when you give it and again when the person shows appreciation. (That's why, when you receive a compliment, you never want to discount it. It deprives the donor of their return gift.)

- *Use compliments.* Compliments are verbal gifts with the same triple rebound of feel-good hormones for you. They are great connectors with other people. They are also great motivators for the Person because they work to override all those immobilizing negatives that their losses cause. Use them often.

When I tell Gordon how well he is eating, he really does eat better! It's the same when I tell him how easy it is to get him out of his chair. He really can get up better! -- Virginia

Don't worry about overdoing the praise. All people react positively to compliments initially—and for the Person, that is the only reaction that counts. They take compliments literally.

Don't forget to compliment yourself too. Make kudos a regular part of your self-talk.

- ***Smile, laugh, nod, giggle.*** Humor is a great healer. But you don't have to be funny. Smiles and even nods work. You don't really need a reason. Just do it. They all trigger your body to respond as though you were saying "Yes! Yes! Yes!" Even looking for reasons to laugh, smile and nod causes your body to respond as though you were actually doing it.

I laugh with Gordon every day. Sometimes we just do something silly like playing patty-cake and laughing about it. I've started nodding to him a lot, mostly for no reason, just to see if it make either of us feel better. Would you believe it does? That really surprised me. -- Virginia

Like Virginia, find something to laugh about with the Person every day. It will not only help both of you feel better, it will add a special feeling of connection with its own positive effect.

- ***Be grateful.*** As with laughter, you don't need a reason to be grateful. Looking for a reason is enough to trigger those feel-good hormones.

Every night just before I go to sleep, I think about what I'm grateful for. I can always find something, even after a difficult day, even if it is only the fact that the day is over and it really helps me relax. -- Virginia

While simply being grateful is enough to trigger your hormones, having a reason increases your good feelings even more. Write these down and read them regularly.

I have a Thanks Jar. When I have something to be grateful about, I write in on a little note and put it in my jar. Then when I feel down, I pull out one of the notes and relive that good moment. -- Virginia

Like other positive behaviors, gratefulness is contagious and so make sure you share. Tell others and give examples.

- **_Slow down._** This is different than taking time to think before you act. Take time to look at the sunsets, notice your loved one's smile, or enjoy a relaxed meal. Even talking slower is better for you. Speedy actions cause the motivation hormones connected with negativity to flow and make you more nervous and uncomfortable.

I've developed the habit of talking slower even when I'm not with Gordon. I used to think it was something I did for him so he'd have time to process. Now I know that it is also good for me. Of course, Gordon is going to reflect my happier, more relaxed mood and that's to my benefit too. -- Virginia

- **_Enjoy contagious happiness and second-hand positivity._** Smile and watch others smile back at you. Laugh with the laugh track on TV. Enjoy positive pictures, movies, photos of past happy events. You don't even need the photo--just daydream about some past joy and you get to relive the same happy feelings.

- **_Play._** Take time to play, to do something you enjoy each day. This is not only a basic need, it is one that triggers those feel-good hormones that make you feel positive.

Gordon and I put puzzles together. It can take us a long time because we don't do a lot at one time but we enjoy it and it's something we have fun doing together. -- Virginia

- **_Be discriminating._** You know to be careful about what the Person watches. But those scary movies and dismal news stories also trigger your own negative responses. Avoid as many as you can to make being and staying positive easier.

***

Responsive Care Takeaways for Being Positive:

- Positive people are happier, healthier and can manage stress better.

- Negative emotions are usually the first ones humans notice and the first to be acted upon.

- Being positive requires taking the time to make conscious choices.

Action: Become aware of negative thoughts and actions.

Action: Take time to consciously choose a more positive way to think and act.

Action: Make consistent small changes replacing the old negative ways with more positive thinking and actions until these become habit.

Actions that help a person stay positive include:

o Treat yourself as a friend and use encouraging self-talk instead of put-downs.

o Remember the five positives to combat one negative rule.

o Give gifts, which provide a triple shot of feel-good hormones and make both you and the giftee feel more positive. Gifts can be of time and thought, not just things.

o Give compliments. These act the same as gifts. They are especially good for the Person who responds to the initial happy feeling and doesn't discriminate.

o Smile, laugh, nod, giggle. All trigger the same positive feelings. No reason needed; just do it!

- Be grateful. The good feeling happens from just BEING grateful. The feelings increase with looking for, sharing or listing reasons to be grateful.
- Slow down your actions and even your words. You'll be less anxious and more relaxed.
- Enjoy contagious happiness and second-hand positivity. You can even daydream and relive the same happy feelings.
- Play and let the feel-good hormones loose!
- Be discriminating: Avoid negative media, people or anything else that will trigger negative feelings.

15. Respite

respite: *A break from a difficult, exhausting or emotionally draining situation.*

caregiver support group: *A place where care partners can share experiences and concerns, build friendships and feel refreshed.*

respite care: *Planned or emergency short-term and time-limited breaks for care partners.*

adult day care: *A program that provides a few hours of supervised care with activities such as meals and socialization one or more times a week.*

***

Care partnering is a stressful job anyway you do it. Even when you get your basic needs met, you are going to have periods of stress. That's where respite comes in. Consider the following suggestions valuable survival tools, not luxuries that you might try if you ever find the time or energy.

Support Groups. There are many excuses for not attending a support group.

I don't want to listen to other people whine.

I don't want to talk about my loved one--it sounds disrespectful.

I don't have time, or the energy.

I'm awfully private, I'd never be able to talk to strangers.

 Or, well, you name it.

But group members tell a different story:

I don't know what I'd have done without my group!

My support group gives me strength to keep on.

I can talk about my loved one here and the group members understand; they've been there. They know my loved one's behavior is dementia-caused, not personal.

I learn new ideas, new ways to do things, new resources. "

I come away from the group feeling stronger. How do caregivers survive without a support group?

The list could go on and on.

Attend a local group if you can. The friends and support you will find there will make it worth the effort. Some groups have free day care for the Person during the meeting. If you can't attend a local group, there are online groups. Find them in the Additional Resource section of this book. The great thing about the online groups is that if you feel a need to vent at three in the morning, you can! Many care partners belong to a local group and an online group as well.

I live in a small community where there isn't a LBD caregivers support group. They do have a dementia caregivers support group but it only meets once a month. The senior center also offers a monthly general caregivers support group. By belonging to both I get to be out with people who understand my isolation and many of my issues twice a month. Then I belong to a LBD online group where I can discuss the stuff that members in the other groups might not understand. -- Ted

Ted is on the right track. Take advantage of what your local community offers and supplement it with one or more online groups if you need to. Of course, even care partners who are fortunate enough to have a local LBD support group often belong to online groups as well. They each have their place.

Respite time. At about the same time the Person can no longer be left alone, the care partner needs to start taking regular respite breaks. You may still feel able to do most of the needed tasks and therefore don't believe you need help. However, you still need occasional "time off." You can't be continually responsible 24/7 and expect to do a good job. The stress frays tempers, causes mistakes and leads to more behaviors from the Person.

Many care teams start a routine of regular visits to adult day care early on.

A bus picks Roger up, takes him to his day club and brings him back. Roger looks forward to going. It is early in his dementia journey but he's begun to feel uncomfortable in regular groups. There he fits right in. They play cards and visit and even have songfests. -- Jackie

Try to start day care visits while the Person can still enjoy socialization, as Roger does. Just as importantly, the Person will also be more likely to be able to understand your need for respite. Let it go until you really need it and your Person will be likely to view the visits as desertion and resist going.

Some facilities treat the Person as a volunteer, asking them to help with various tasks.

Larry was a workaholic before he retired. The day care staff recognized that and told him they needed a volunteer to help with setting up the tables for playing cards and putting everything away later. He loves his Day Club days and can't wait for the bus to come and take him to the center! -- Doris

Larry gets to feel a bit like he used to when he felt needed at his job. This can greatly increase a Person's desire to attend.

Responsive Care Takeaways for Respite:

- Support groups provide a care partner with a place to share, learn, vent and relate with others having similar issues.

Action: Consider a support group a necessary part of the caregiving job.

- Support groups can be local or online, general or specific to a certain disease. Each has its value.

Action: Find and join a local group with the best fit and supplement it with online groups as needed or wanted.

- A care partner needs regular respite time to keep burnout at bay.

Action: Start respite care early so that the Person can adjust to it while change is still tolerable.

Action: Use adult day care as a socialization time for the Person and a respite time for the care partner.

Section Three: Providing the Care

The previous chapters have been about gaining knowledge:

- Information from senses is identified by concrete thinking, picks up an emotion, and is processed by abstract thinking.

- Abstract thinking requires executive skills, which tend to fade early with LBD and later with other dementias.

- Concrete thinking remains: literal, impulsive, single-minded, inflexible, current, without empathy, based on initial information and closely connected to emotions.

- Emotions also remain. The initial emotion attached to new information is likely to be residual and negative.

- Negative emotions are motivators, driving a person into action and often precipitating behaviors.

- Positive emotions are calming, encouraging one to stay and enjoy the pleasantness, with less need for behaviors.

- Stress is an overload of physical, mental or emotional pressure/tension, along with negative feelings.

- A Person has a very low stress threshold. Common dementia-related physical problems decrease it even further.

- Decreasing negative feelings and stress results in fewer behaviors and psychological symptoms of dementia.

- Alternative options for behavior management should always be tried first.

- Behavior management drugs may have serious side effects and should be used only after alternative options alone have been tried and failed.

- When used in combination with alternative options, behavior management drugs are usually more effective in lower doses than when used alone.

- The Person deserves a care partner who is as physically, emotionally and mentally healthy as possible.

- Improv acting has a lot in common with dementia caregiving. It provides a way for care partners to feel more comfortable accepting and flowing with the Person's reality.

- A care partner needs to be flexible enough to let go of what doesn't work and move on, without guilt and self-blame.

The next chapters are about putting this knowledge into practice:

- Utilizing knowledge about the brain, emotions, stress and self-care to choose effective behaviors and words.

- Viewing the job as a team activity. The Person is encouraged to see themselves as an active participant in their care, rather than a passive care receiver. Likewise, the care partner doesn't try to do their part of the job alone.

- Recognizing the Person as someone with unique likes, dislikes and needs.

- Using empathy to see from the Person's point of view.

- Accepting the Person's reality and joining it enough to replace negative feelings with positive ones.

- Engaging the Person in ways that preserve respect and keep communication open.

- Exploring the many alternative treatment options and using those that are appropriate.

16. Being a Team

team member: *One of at least two people who are working together towards a common goal.*

***

When caregivers redefine themselves as care partners, they acknowledge that living with dementia is a team activity, with at least two team members, the care *partner* and the **Person**. In a previous book, we stated.

The person living with dementia and the caregiver are a team. While only one has the symptoms, both are affected. Married couple, parent and adult child, siblings or any other caregiver arrangement, the pair are partners in this endeavor. -- Managing Cognitive Issues

Even before the Person loses their ability to initiate, plan and do most daily living activities, apathy can be present. Thus the care partner may be thrust into the leadership role even before it seems necessary.

Family members continually report that even Persons who are still able to read well are seldom interested in reading about their disorder. They prefer to let their care partners do the research. Thus, it will usually be up to the care partner to read, sift and share information as the Person can tolerate or wishes to hear. --Managing Cognitive Issues

As dementia takes its toll and abilities fail, feeling like a useful team member becomes more difficult for the Person. Balancing the checkbook becomes a puzzle, driving a car becomes a danger and so on. Each loss adds more feelings of inadequacy, frustration and lack of empowerment.

These losses also add confusion and emotional pain when the Person's waning abilities also prevent an understanding that there is even a problem.

Mason still thinks he can drive just fine. Trying to get him to accept that he needs to let me drive has been a difficult task. "He accuses me of treating him like a child and says that he feels useless. -- Iris

Iris felt she had to begin taking responsibility for many of the things that Mason used to do well. Mason can't understand the need for this and sees it not as support, but as an attack on his manhood. His resistance increases the stress she already feels from having to take on these new jobs.

By being responsive to Mason's underlying emotions, Iris can validate them so that he feels heard. Then she can use his still intact abilities to help him accept his limitations and find other ways to feel useful and active.

Iris can use Mason's fading memory and attention span to help him accept the loss of valued tasks. For example, she can do the bills when he isn't around.

When Mason complains about lost team responsibilities, such as driving the car, validating his negative feelings will take away much of the anger. "It's really frustrating isn't it?" Then Iris can distract him by asking for help with a task such as vacuuming, that he can still do.

I've had to take over our finances too. Mason was making awful errors and spending money we didn't have. But this had always been his job. I'm afraid I'll be just as bad as Mason! -- Iris

If, like Iris, you aren't used to handing the family finances or any other task you must assume, get guidance from an expert.

It's better to spend some time and money now than to risk making major mistakes later. Iris may be able to do just fine after someone shows her what she needs to do. Ask your bank or the local Area Agency on Aging for resources for this kind of help.

Leaders and followers. Teams include leaders or initiators and followers. Dementia takes away a Person's ability to initiate or lead, but they can often express their wishes and emotions with nonverbal cues. Leading the team becomes the care partner's job. It can involve figuring out what the Person feels, needs or wants, initiating the action, helping the Person to feel included and mirroring the behavior for them to reflect.

Mason likes to go walking, but he doesn't suggest it anymore. He may get agitated and then I know he wants something. If ask him what is bothering him, he can't tell me. But if I ask if he'd like to go for a walk, he's always ready to go. -- Iris

Mason is past the stage where he initiates actions or asks verbally for help. Iris uses what she knows about Mason to guess what he wants. Then she offers an invitation that moves the action on.

Invitations require little processing. Questions about what is wrong or even a suggestion would require processing that could make Mason confused, frustrated and stuck.

Sometimes it takes a long time for Mason to decide. I've learned to stay quiet and be patient. -- Iris

Even invitations can sometimes take time to process. Persons are very attuned to their care partner's feelings. When Iris stays patient and positive, Mason can mirror her relaxed attitude.

Mason is much more likely to go along with what I want if I tell him what's going to happen. -- Iris

Clueing Mason in on what's about to happen makes him feel a part of the team. It also adds security so that he feels more relaxed. However, Iris only talks about what is going to happen in the near future. If she gets too far in the future, she'll cause Mason to become anxious.

It also helps if he knows I'm going to be doing it with him. -- Iris

If Iris isn't involved in the task, Mason loses the "team" feeling-and the sense of security that belonging brings. Yes, team members can work separately, but knowing that requires abstract thinking. For Mason, if Iris isn't there it isn't a team!

Making family decisions is another adult task where the Person can feel slighted. Although the Person's failing thinking abilities makes this a difficult, often unsafe task, they can still be consulted. Being asked for their opinion makes a Person feel more useful, needed, valued and empowered.

Decisions are mostly up to me now, but I still consult Mason about important stuff. I told him, "Let's sell the brown car. We don't use it anymore and we need the money." He shrugged and said, "OK, if that's what you want to do." Because I know how Mason hated to stop driving, I was really glad to accept his permission to sell, albeit reluctant. -- Iris

Iris tried to ease Mason's pain about the loss of his car by framing her suggestion as an invitation that prompted an affirmative answer. It worked; agreeing with Iris allowed Mason to feel part of the decision-making team and gave him a feeling of control that made letting the car go less painful. She also didn't say the car was Mason's although he had been the primary driver, another way to decrease Mason's grief.

156

Mason was surprised when our son took the car to a dealer; he didn't remember our conversation, but he didn't get angry, thank goodness. -- Iris

Although Mason had forgotten the discussion, he still had residual positive feelings about being consulted and an emotional memory of his release of the car. If Iris had sold the car without discussing it with Mason, he might have been quite angry. As it was, his residual feelings made acceptance more possible.

Even though he didn't get angry, Mason was depressed and sad about the loss of his car. I gave him a hug and told him how sorry I was. It seemed to help. -- Iris

It is always a temptation to ignore a Person's negative feelings, hoping that they will go away. Instead, like Iris, acknowledge and validate them, making it easier for the Person to let them go.

Residential Care Issue. As a Person's ability to recognize family wanes, care partners sometimes think they are no longer needed. Even in a facility where there is a good staff-resident ratio, the family care partner is a vital team member.

I've seen situations where a caregiver with five mobile and continent residents one day had three incontinent residents with one in a wheelchair the next or flu can make all five residents incontinent. Families of residents need to show up often enough to be available and able to help in such situations and to advocate for changes if they are needed. -- Connie, memory care volunteer

Family can find it painful to visit a loved one who no longer remembers them, but it remains highly important. A resident who has regular family visits will almost always get better care.

***

Responsive Care Takeaways for Being a Team.

- Living with dementia is a team activity with both care partner and Person having active roles.

- These roles change over time, with the care partner taking on tasks the Person can no longer do safely or correctly.

- While the Person may give up many tasks willingly, they may view the loss of some as attacks on their adulthood.

  Attitude: Practice being patient with an empathetic awareness of the Person's feelings of loss and disenfranchisement.

  Actions:

  o Keep reminders of these losses out of sight.

  o Expect, encourage and validate vented feelings about losses due to decreased abilities.

  o Ask the Person to help with tasks they can still do.

  Self-care: Seek guidance from an expert for any task you had to take over that you feel unready to handle.

  Actions:

  o Including the Person as a part of the team causes positive feelings of being needed, valued and empowered.

  o A Person cannot initiate but they can follow.

  Attitude: Practice positive collaboration and togetherness, which the Person can mirror.

  Actions:

  o Make guesses about unvoiced wishes using nonverbal cues and a knowledge of their likes and dislikes.

  o Identify the task as a team effort.

  o Share what is going to happen in the near future.

- Having one's opinion consulted about family decisions helps the Person to feel like a part of the decision-making team.

- An agreement that the action is needed will work to dilute negative feelings when it happens.

  Actions:

  o Frame the suggestion to elicit an agreement.

  o Validate any negative feelings that still surround the event when it happens.

- A care partner's job doesn't end even when the Person doesn't know them.

17. Being Person-Centered

person-centered: *Respectful of and responsive to an individual's preferences, needs, and values.*

Person (with a capital P): *The Person living with dementia.*

person: *Anyone. They may or may not be living with dementia.*

***

Saying "Person(s) *living* with dementia" helps one to recognize that the Person is living *with* the disease, but is not the disease itself. Dementia care works best that way--when the Person is recognized as an adult person, not as a disease, a task or a child.

The Best Friends^{TM} Dementia Bill of Rights[27] is developed from many interviews with a variety of people with dementia. It says that every Person diagnosed with dementia deserves:

- To be informed of one's diagnosis

- To have appropriate, ongoing medical care

- To be treated as an adult, listened to, and afforded respect for one's feelings and point of view

- To be with individuals who know one's life story, including cultural and spiritual traditions

- To experience meaningful engagement throughout the day

- To live in a safe and stimulating environment

- To be outdoors on a regular basis

- To be free from psychotropic medications whenever possible

- To have welcomed physical contact, including hugging, caressing, and handholding

- To be an advocate for oneself and for others

- To be part of a local, global or online community

- To have care partners well trained in dementia care

While most care partners make an effort to respect these rights, there are many ways to get off track. In our disease-centered medical system, the actual person involved can get overlooked. When a care partner has a lot to do, getting the task done can become more important than the person. Drugs are sometimes used as shortcuts to behavior management when more person-centered alternative options might work as well or at least decrease the amount of drugs needed to do the job. As a Person living with dementia needs more care and guidance, it is easy to relegate them to a child-like status.

A waning ability to speak and/or act for oneself brings about feelings of loss of personhood, of "Who I Am." In a care facility, these feelings increase as the Person becomes one of many. With all of these and more, feelings of being misunderstood, unwanted, unneeded, unlovable and unloved increase and generate an even greater likelihood of behaviors.

Still present abilities. A care partner who is aware of a Person's remaining abilities, can respond in encouraging ways, find alternative methods of communicating, and help the Person feel useful, needed, and loved.

My mother-in-law Lois was adamant that she would talk to the doctor and that I was to stay silent. I tried to do as she demanded, but her fractured sentences and gestures, easily understood by me, were unintelligible to the doctor. When I finally tried to interpret, Lois became furious. -- Sue

Feeling the loss of her autonomy and personhood, Lois was trying to do what she once did well. Sue tried to support her but ended up making Lois feel more inept--and angry. Sue's concern about a wasted doctor's visit if Lois wasn't able to be clear was valid. But so was Lois's need to be her own person.

After a few false starts, we hit on a solution. I told Lois I liked to take a list with me so that I'd remember everything I wanted to tell the doctor. She agreed that this might be a good idea for her too and so that's what we did. -- Sue

When Sue admitted a need for memory boosts, this made it easier for Lois to accept her own need and still feel "normal."

At first Lois made the list out but now I do it for her, being very careful to use her words even if they don't make much sense. Then, with her permission, I make a copy "for her records." Lois puts the original in her purse "to give to the doctor." -- Sue

Sue let Lois do as much of the task as she could and even when Sue had to take it over, she "followed directions."

Since others couldn't always understand Lois's lists, I make another copy, with interpretations as needed, for the nurse or in some cases, to email directly to the doctor. -- Sue

Sue met the need to provide the doctor with good information by making and delivering an interpreted copy of Lois's list but doing it in such a way that Lois didn't feel discounted.

The result was that Lois gets to feel independent while the doctor understands her needs. -- Sue

The time Sue took to prepare paved the way for Lois to feel independent while getting her needs met. It can take creativity and more than one try to meet both physical and emotional needs. However, the joy of a Person who feels both independent and understood is usually reflected in fewer behaviors. For instance, Lois became less demanding in the doctor's office.

Lois still saw herself as the person she always was--and in many ways she still was. She still had the same likes, dislikes and many of the same needs as well as some new ones that she may not understand well. Sue had known Lois for 20 years, but even then using the Life Story Questionnaire[28] can add helpful information.

Completing this form can be a fun activity, with memories of past events. To fill out the form for Lois, Sue asked questions of her husband and other family members as well as Lois. Each added shared stories and information. Even if you know your loved one well, take the time to complete this form with for later, when others may need it.

Triggers for stress. Likes and dislikes vary and so do stressors. By being aware of the Person-specific conditions that trigger stress, the care partner can avert many stressful situations.

Ken has developed a fear of the color red. Anytime I wear red, he gets combative and so of course, I don't wear anything red anymore. But its more than that. I bought red dishes because I'd heard that they were easier for people living with dementia to use but when I use them, he thinks his

food is poisoned. Needless to say, they stay stored away! --
Kathy

Anything perceived as bothersome, annoying, threatening, or disrupting will trigger negative feelings. Allowed to continue unaddressed, these will almost always result in stress-related behaviors. Once you know the triggers, you can make changes to remove or decrease them.

***

Responsive Care Takeaways for Being Person-Centered:

- Persons living with dementia are people with feelings, needs, likes and dislikes, people who still see themselves as independent, useful and functional adults.

  ### *Attitudes:*

  o Acceptance of the Person as they are.
  o Empathy for their need to feel independent, useful and worthy of love.
  o Respectful of the Person's need to be treated as an adult even as abilities and emotions make them more child-like.
  o Awareness of those things most likely to act as a Person's stressors.

Actions:

o Encourage still-present abilities and find alternate methods to deal with fading ones.

o Take time, creativity and effort to find "work-arounds," that meet a Person's needs for autonomy while maintaining adequate care.

o Complete the Life Story Questionnaire early on to help care facilities provide person-centered care in the future.

o Identify and act to decrease or remove stressors.

18. Being Accepting

acceptance: *Voluntary and intentional attitude, aimed at utility and function rather than truth.*

belief: *Based on what one considers to be fact or truth.*

accept: *To agree to a situation as is, without protest or attempting to change it. One can accept with or without believing.*

***

Accept that dementia changes abilities. Dementia is a progressive disease and the journey is one of continual change. Dementia changes a Person's ability to do things such as drive, handle money or tell time. Each of these changes requires the care partner to recognize them, accept them, and make corresponding changes in their own actions.

Recognition isn't always easy. Because the journey is so gradual, changes can sneak up. A Person doesn't stop being able to do something all at once.

I really don't like to drive, but Steve's not safe anymore. It took me a while to realize this. I knew he was getting slower but I still thought he was safe. But the last time he drove, he went right through a stop sign. I'm doing the driving now. – Rhonda

Rhonda recognized that Steve's driving was getting worse, but she wasn't willing to accept that it was unsafe until he did something that was hard to ignore. This is normal for care partners everywhere. We don't want to accept that dementia is eroding useful functions like driving, especially when it means making unwelcome changes of our own.

Don has always gone walking but now he gets lost. He can't understand why I don't want him to go alone and so if I'm busy, he just sneaks out. -- Darlene

Dementia changes the Person's abilities to think and respond. Rhonda was fortunate that she was able to take over the driving so easily. Darlene's case is more common, where Don doesn't understand why he can't continue to do what he has always done. Without abstract thinking, the Person can no longer judge when something they've always done is now unsafe.

Accept that the Person's reality changes. With an understanding of the connection between residual negative feelings and a Person's apparently irrational conclusions, it is easier to accept their new reality. With an understanding of the firmness of these conclusions, it is easier to accept the resulting dramas as unchangeable. When you accept that, it becomes easier to let go of your own reality and accept theirs.

If this is still difficult for you, try improv. Consider yourself an actor in a drama where the Person has set the scene and your job is to play it out.

We've always had a very honest relationship. We've never lied to each other. That's why these changes in Gerry's behavior were so difficult for me to deal with. I understood that if I played along, he would be less agitated, but it just felt wrong. Now I pretend I'm an improv actor and follow his lead. -- Olivia

As the Person changes, so must your responses. It is not only futile but detrimental to try to reason with someone who can't reason.

Let go of old expectations. When expectations are no longer valid, they block communication. Instead, accept what is. You don't have to like what is happening, not in the moment and not with the disease. Nor do you have to believe, although you must suspend your disbelief enough to avoid expressing or acting upon it. With acceptance, you and the Person can move away from the pain and the resulting behaviors and into a place where supportive communication is possible.

At first, Carol believed me when I told her that the children she saw weren't real. Now, she gets mad even when I tell her, "I know you see them but I don't." Last time she told me, "You think I'm crazy. But I'm not. Those kids live right there in the closet." -- Harold

Harold can't accept that Carol's dementia has progressed to where her belief in what she sees is non-negotiable.

The kids don't really bother Carol. What does upset her is that I can't accept them as real. But I can't. I don't see them. I know they aren't there. How is that supportive of her to let her go on thinking they are?

Harold is still clinging to the idea that somehow he can help Carol be the way she used to be before her hallucinations. That ship has sailed and he is stuck on shore with his old expectations. Harold needs to learn that accepting Carol's reality is not "letting her" do anything. She is going to believe her reality no matter what Harold does. He can't change that. He can only change the way he responds.

All this talk about accepting her reality just sounds like fancy words for lying to me. How can I treat my wife that way? -- Harold

Harold's belief about lying is also faulty. Yes, in his world view, accepting the presence of the children is lying. However, in the reality that Carol is stuck with, she'd be lying if she agreed that the children weren't there. In this impasse, only Harold has the ability to change.

Letting go of old expectations is especially difficult for care partners like Harold who have lived with their loved ones for many years and developed a history of mutual beliefs. "We never lied to each other" is the way things were. Now dementia has changed the rules and Harold must also change if he is going to be a successful care partner.

Accept that there are no hard, fast rules. Dementia changes some rules for everyone, such as the need to let go of old expectations and the need to enter the Person's reality if you want successful communication.

However, many changes are individual. What works for one may not for another. While there are many similarities in the way a Person thinks and acts, triggers for both negative and positive emotions will be different. A good share of a care partner's expertise is in knowing "what works and what doesn't" for their specific loved one. Also, be aware that this can change as the dementia progresses.

The progress of a Person's dementia also changes the way they respond to behavior management drugs. In Chapter 2- Drugs and Drug Sensitivity, support group members discussed the way each of their loved ones reacted differently to similar drugs. This sensitivity tends to increase with time and so it continues to be trial and error. It never stops changing because dementia keeps changing the rules.

Accept that the present moment is the only one that counts. There is no yesterday or tomorrow, there is only now. Telling the Person that you've never lied to them or that you'll take them out for ice cream tomorrow doesn't work anymore. Only the present matters.

When my mom, was in a nursing home, someone in our family tried to visit her at least every other day. However, she always told me that no one has been to see her in weeks. We put up a calendar and signed in whenever we visited. This helped us to know who had visited and when, but Mom still insisted that she wasn't getting any visitors. – Edith, daughter of Myrtle

Myrtle's dementia had left her with only the present time. She couldn't remember the recent past and the future was equally unreal to her. All Edith and her family could do was give her lots of positive experiences when they did visit so that she'd have positive emotional memories to help her over the loneliness she felt the rest of the time.

***

Responsive Care Takeaways for Being Accepting:

- Dementia changes the rules because it changes the Person's view of reality.

- A Person's dementia will progress so that old expectations and old ways of relating will not work anymore.

- The Person often still feels functional and rational.

- Changes are gradual. Care partners can also have difficulty recognizing and then accepting the changes.

- Effective interactions require an acceptance, but not a belief of the Person's unchangeable "truth."

Attitudes:

- o Open to letting go of old expectations.

- o Open to finding and using new ways to relate.

- o Open to the idea that you are the only one on the team who can change.

Actions:

- o Put your view of reality on hold (it is still your truth, simply suspended) and accept the Person's.

- o Be alert for residual feelings that increase the Person's behavior.

- o Use improv acting to accept the Person's reality, validate negative feelings and move the action in the desired direction.

- o Avoid responses that cause strong, uncomfortable negative emotions.

- o Find and use actions that make positive emotions strong enough to provide comfort and solace.

19. Working with Present Abilities

Dementia takes away many of a Person's skills and limits others. However, not all abilities are lost. Certain skills tend to last longer than others. As you identify what these are and use them, communication will improve and frustrations will decrease, with an accompanying decrease in behaviors.

Thinking. Dementia doesn't happen all at once. A Person will continue to have many of their abilities for a long time. Even those that fade don't leave entirely. Thinking is an example of this. Even late in the journey, a Person's brain still processes what the five senses deliver, but it gets slower, more concrete and less accurate with time.

Use patience and simplicity. When interacting with a Person, taking lots of time and using simple easy to understand (concrete) words will help them use the thinking abilities they have left.

Brian was an English professor but as his dementia advanced, I found that he used simpler words, like "thing" for words he could no longer remember. However, if I got too basic, he'd get mad at me and accuse me of treating him like a child. – Molly

Comprehension often outlasts language abilities, so that Brian will understand what Molly is talking about long after he can talk about it himself, although it may take him a while to process what she says. This is where time is more important than simplicity, especially at first, when cognition is still present but slower.

Maintain continuity. Anything that interferes with the flow of thought will make it more difficult. Interrupting, offering too much information at once, being unclear, or being impatient or irritable can all block the Person's ability to use their remaining abilities.

(Learn more about helpful ways to interact in Chapter 21- Being Engaging.)

Rhythm and music. Rhythm and music travel to the brain on a different path than language does and lasts well into the disease. Rhythm can be especially helpful in facilitating movement and music can improve clarity for hours after it is no longer present. Their path is also very connected to that of emotions so that they can stimulate a variety of emotions, from sadness to happiness. They can also energize or relax. See more in the sections on Music and Rhythm in Chapter 27, Using the Sense Pathways.

Emotions. As thinking abilities fade, emotions take up the slack. They begin to rule the Person's outlook on life and their behavior. Emotions can last long after the reason for them is forgotten. The stronger they are, the longer they last. This can help or harm not only present interactions, but following ones. Positive emotions encourage feelings of security, comfort, happiness and fewer behaviors. Negative emotions tend to be strong and agitating with feelings of fear, anger, discomfort and more behaviors.

Maintain a calm, pleasant attitude. The Person will pick up your emotions and mirror them back to you as behaviors even when your feelings don't pertain to the present interaction. Put your negative emotions on hold until away from your Person.

Monitor your intensity. Even if you are being positive, avoid being too intense. This can be seen as negative and may even imply danger.

Monitor the Person's intensity. Early on, its level of force shows the strength of negative feelings such as frustration, pain or fear. As the ability to judge one's severity of discomfort fades, even minor irritations may be seen as extreme.

Use aligning with emotions as a defusing tool. The one time a care person might want to show some intensity is when attempting to defuse a situation.

My mom got all upset with me when I was trying to brush her hair and started screaming that I was trying to kill her. Anna, the aide came in and tried to calm her down but that only made her worse. A male tech came in and held her down while we waited for the nurse to come with medication. Then when Linda, the nurse did come, she didn't bring a shot. Instead, she yelled at us and shooed us all out of the room. – Shirley, daughter of Beth

Linda aligned with Beth's anger and by removing her perceived threat, became her rescuer. Linda's actions told Beth that she was on her side, that she could trust her.

From around the corner, I could see Mom almost wilt with relief. Then Linda changed to a softer voice and asked Mom what happened. When Mom started telling her about how awful we'd all been, Linda listened and said stuff like "Oh, you poor dear." Linda did some deep breathing and before long, Mom was acting normal. -- Shirley, daughter of Beth

Once Beth felt safe, she was able to stop her defensive battling and respond to Linda's calming efforts. Without the building of trust, Beth would have continued to feel attacked and it wouldn't have worked.

Once Mom was relaxed, Linda said, "I'll bet you are really tired. Would you like to take a little nap?" At Mom's nod, she added, "How about we get Anna in here to help you up on the bed?" Mom nodded again and even smiled! -- Shirley, daughter of Beth

Linda used a technique taught by Teepa Snow, where she aligned with Beth's emotions and became her champion.[29] This calmed Beth down to where she could function normally enough to cooperate. It is a multi-step process:

a) **Align with the Person's anger.** You understand; you are upset too. Make your level of intensity a little less than theirs; you want to de-escalate the situation, not make it worse. (Stay safe. Never get close enough to touch an angry Person.)

b) **Align with the Person's feeling of being a rescued victim.** Kneel at eye-level and croon sympathetic statements. Use touch only when they show a willingness for it, as when they take your offered hand.

c) **Start deep breathing.** The Person will mirror you and this will relax both of you. Now they are aligning with you.

d) **Align with the Person's need to take everything slowly.** Speed tends to feel threatening and can re-escalate the situation.

e) **Align with the Person's need to feel in control.** Once the Person is calmer, include them in the problem solving by wording what you need done as an invitation.

Responsive Care Takeaways for Working with Present Abilities:

- Thinking gets slower, more concrete and more difficult.

  Attitude: Be patient and respectful.

  Action: Use concrete words and phrases. Avoid anything that would interrupt the thought process.

- Rhythm and music travel to the brain on a different, simpler path than language does.

  Action: Use rhythm and music to facilitate movement and improve clarity.

- Emotions last and can help or damage present and future interactions. Intensity fades but can still be identified in others--and viewed as negative even in positive situations.

- Interactions will likely fail unless negative emotions are recognized and verified.

  Attitude: Maintain a calm, pleasant and accepting attitude that the Person can mirror and avoid showing intense emotions.

  Action: Start an interaction with an upset Person by aligning with their negative emotions to validate them and build trust.

20. Being Empathetic

empathy: A two part process of experiencing an event from another's viewpoint while knowing that what you feel is what you would feel in that situation, not what you feel personally.

***

Once you accept the Person's losses, their still-present abilities and their reality, your next step is to empathize. That is, you imagine yourself in their situation with their abilities and think about how you would feel. When a care partner accepts and has empathy for a Person's limitations and views, interactions become less adversarial and stressful. However, empathy isn't always a skill that comes naturally.

Beth: That new aide stole my slippers.

Shirley: I'll bet there just right here somewhere, Mom. Ah, see! They were under the bed where you couldn't see them.

Beth: Shirley, I tell you she stole them. I know she did. Those aren't mine. Take them away.

Shirley: But Mom,....

Shirley is stuck with her expectations of how her mother used to be, pre-dementia.

Mom was always the most generous, thoughtful person but not anymore and nothing I do makes a difference. -- Shirley

With empathy, Shirley could see her mother's behavior as it is now and not as painfully lacking in the way she wants it to be.

So how can Shirley learn to be empathetic?

Have the knowledge. It helps to know how the Person's brain is changing the rules. Beth sees life differently now. This is not on purpose but because the disease makes it different. She sees life concretely, with her residual fears as guides. Her slippers are there or if not, she fears that they are stolen—and therefore they ARE stolen.

The change that Shirley needs to remember is that her mother is no longer capable of empathy. This takes abstract thinking. She can see only from her own perspective, her own reality.

Accept the changes. Just knowing that dementia changes the rules isn't enough. Shirley has to make it personal by accepting that her mother has advanced to where this information is true for her. This step from intellectual knowledge to personal acceptance can be a difficult, sometimes heart-wrenching move, but it must be made if you are to have successful interactions.

Experience their reality. Using what she's learned, Shirley can now imagine herself in Beth's place, see the situation from Beth's point of view and enter Beth's reality.

Here's what might happen if Shirley used empathy instead of reason:

Beth: I can't find my slippers. The new aide stole them. I just know she did.

Shirley: Oh, Mom. I know how you loved those slippers. (showing empathy)

Beth: Yes, and now they are gone. The aide took them. (Beth felt heard and didn't feel a need to get angrier.)

Shirley: Tell you what Mom. I'll get you some more. (Shirley didn't try to tell her mom a different reality...that she'd found the slippers under the bed.)

Beth: I don't want different ones. I want those. You find that aide and take them back from her.

Shirley: OK, Mom, I'll work on that. (She can leave and come back into the room with the slippers, saying something like, "I got them for you, Mom." Since the event was never allowed to escalate, Beth is likely to forget it once the situation is resolved, especially if Shirley changes the subject right away.)

Look for the feelings. Often the drama is more about the Person's feelings than it is about the situation.

When Larry first accused me of planning to run away with our neighbor, I was shocked. Ben and his wife have been our good friends for years. That would be the last thing I'd do! -- Doris

At first, Doris took Larry's words at face value. Then with empathy, she can move past the words and consider how she'd feel in that same.

"In Larry's place, I might think that I was so helpless and worthless that no one would want to stay with me. Then I'd really be frightened. How would I survive if my care partner left?" -- Doris

In the moment. For the Person, there is only the present reality. Like Beth's *suspicion* that her slippers *might have been* stolen became the actual theft in her mind, Larry's FEAR of abandonment becomes BEING abandoned in his mind. With no reasoning interface between the fear and the conclusion, the fear becomes the fact.

Limit fear of abandonment by increasing the Person's self-worth with regular expressions of appreciation and affection.

181

I've found that if I continually show Larry how much I like having him around, he is less likely to make these awful accusations. I try to be positive around him all the time. I give him lots of hugs and little back rubs. I tell him how much he means to me so often I must sound like a broken record. -- Doris

For a normal person, it takes at least five positives to offset one negative interaction. For the Person living with dementia, the number is going to be much higher. You just can't do this too much, even if it feels exaggerated to you. The positive feelings from these interactions last even when the memory of them does not.

Opportunities for the use of empathy occur every day and in many different situations. Imagine that:

- You are in a crowd and your slow thinking causes you to have difficulty sifting out all the action and making sense of it.

Would you feel overwhelmed, nervous or ineffective?

- Someone brushes by you and your poor peripheral vision makes that feel like an attack.

Would you feel scared, angry or defensive?

- Without impulse control, you hit out in self-defense.

Would you have difficulty understanding why others are upset with you for defending yourself?

- Your care partner insists that you weren't being attacked when in your mind, you clearly were.

Would you feel angry, betrayed, abandoned or hurt?

- You are trying to say something and you can't make anyone understand or accept your words.

Would you feel frustrated and angry?

In each of the above situations, the Person would experience feelings like those mentioned. If you realize that this is happening, you can defuse the situation by responding with words and actions directed towards the feelings rather than Person's behaviors. Such modifications in your behavior will allow the Person to feel safer, less frustrated and more comfortable, with fewer behaviors.

Knowing the "why" of their behavior really helps a care partner's ability to accept and empathize. It is common nature to want to cling to your own reality. The change to recognizing and then accepting the Person's reality doesn't occur all at once. Just keep trying.

With support group members or willing friends, try role playing. This is a great way to help you get a feel for what it is like to be a Person living with dementia. Take turns being the Person and then the care partner during some common interactions. Do the interactions with and without empathy. That is, as though you don't know anything about how the dementia brain works and then as though you do. Then talk about the feelings that both of you had during each of the interactions. What was the most frustrating? What felt best?

Empathy helps you to avoid taking the Person's apparently irrational actions personally. When you have a better understanding of the Person's view, it is easier to see past the painful words and behaviors to the underlying disease that is the real culprit.

***

Responsive Care Takeaways for Being Empathetic:

- With empathy you experience the same emotions you think another would feel about a situation.

  ### *Attitudes:*

  o Accept that the Person's reality is the only one that matters.

  o Understand that the Person's feelings drive their actions.

  o Accept that the Person's only time is now.

  ### *Actions:*

  o Imagine how you'd feel in their situation, believing as they do. Respond to those feelings in the Person.

  o Look past the drama to find the feelings and respond to them instead of the voiced complaint.

  o Use positive words and actions regularly to decrease the appearance of behaviors.

  ### *Self-care:*

  o Practice empathetic responses with other care partners or support group members to make it easier to avoid getting caught up in old actions and hurt feelings with your Person.

  o Use a support group for venting and releasing hurt feelings you may still have.

  o Do your research. When you know that it is the disorder and not the Person talking, it is easier to do what you need to do to accept and defuse a hurtful behavior.

184

21. Being Engaging

to engage: *to occupy, attract or involve someone's interest*

communication: *a two-way process of interaction, where information, ideas and feelings are exchanged.*

mindful listening: *Listening with eyes, ears, touch and empathy. Being aware of the whole Person and looking past their behaviors to discover the original message.*

empathetic responding: *Responding to a Person in ways they can hear and accept.*

nonverbal cues: *Gestures, facial expressions and even dementia-related behaviors used to express needs and wishes.*

***

As dementia progresses, communication becomes more difficult because thinking is slower, abstract thinking is lost and language skills degenerate. Mindful listening and responding, acceptance, patience, clarity, simplicity and nonverbal cues all become important communication tools.

Mindful Listening

To have a successful conversation with a Person, start by listening mindfully, with your full attention.

Listen with your knowledge. Behaviors usually follow other less extreme but unsuccessful efforts to communicate.

Carol will start rubbing the arms of her wheelchair when she is getting frustrated. That's when I know she's trying to tell me something and I'm not understanding what it is. -- Harold

Carol's behavior may be:

- An expression of frustration at her inability to get the message across.
- Fueled by underlying residual emotions triggered by a current event.
- Triggered more directly by something painful or uncomfortable that she is experiencing but cannot identify.

It can be any combination of the three. If Carol is uncomfortable because of something she can't explain, it is likely to trigger residual emotions. Then, if Harold can't understand what she wants, she's going to be frustrated.

Stay calm and pleasant. The first step in successful engagement is to avoid negative emotions. These usually strong emotions demand the Person's attention and draw their focus away from an increasingly difficult ability to communicate verbally.

- Pay close attention, using empathy to understand and relate.
- Use your acceptance skills to maintain a positive environment and avoid any disagreement.

Listen carefully. As verbal skills fade, the Person turns to other forms of communication. Even if the Person knows what they want to say, their inability to make one's needs and wishes known can be extremely frustrating. These strong emotions and accompanying behaviors often cover up the original message.

- Look for nonverbal cues with all of your senses.
- Listen for emotional cues too.

Be aware of underlying residual emotions. These trigger the Person's apparently irrational behaviors. For example, a general feeling of loss may result in the idea of theft and a loss of self-worth often fosters fears of abandonment. Other residual emotions are more individual.

Gerry almost drowned as a child and he's been afraid of water ever since. He used to be able to take showers just fine but since his dementia got worse, getting him to take a shower is too stressful for both of us. I just give him bed-baths. -- Olivia

When Gerry was able to use abstract thinking, he knew that showers were safe. Now they are fearful events that must be avoided. Olivia used her knowledge of Gerry and his illness to look past his behaviors and recognize the residual emotions that caused them. Then she adjusted her response to trigger fewer of these emotions.

Be alert for nonverbal cues. Facial expressions, hand gestures, general body movements and even at times, dementia-related behaviors are often more accurate cues than words that have become garbled. Nonverbal cues don't require the symbolic interpretation that words do and are therefore easier for the brain to process. As language skills fade the Person will turn to these more and more.

Be a language detective. As your Person's language skills degenerate, words become lost…the "it's on the tip of my tongue" syndrome. Inaccurate words may be substituted, often unconsciously, such as words in the same group (green for blue), rhyming words (glue for blue), words starting with the same letter (big for blue) or even with no connection at all.

- Use mindful listening and nonverbal cues to figure out what your Person really means.

- A mutual history is also a great help. If you don't have a mutual history, learn from those who do have one with the Person.

Be alert for irritants that the Person may not be able to identify. Behaviors may appear when the Person's body attempts to express needs not consciously recognized, as when increased behaviors herald a urinary tract infection. The pain and discomfort from such physical irritations take priority in the Person's brain, moving their already limited focus away from actual communication. This results in an even poorer ability to verbalize.

- Look past the behaviors for unconscious cues such as limping or cradling a possibly sore abdomen.
- View the behaviors themselves as possible early cues of internal distress such as a urinary tract infection.

Be accepting. Once you've listened mindfully, accepting what your Person offers you without resistance will move the conversation forward in a way that trying to reorient can't.

Empathetic Responding

When you can put yourself in the Person's place, it is easier to respond to what you pick up with mindful listening in ways they can hear and accept.

Work with present abilities. (See Chapter 19 -Working with Present Abilities) This means taking your time, using simplicity, clarity and staying in the moment.

Take your time. Processing has become hard work for your Person. Their brain processes very slowly, one thought at a time.

- Be cheerfully patient and relaxed. Forced patience is as uncomfortable as rushing.

188

- Talk slowly in a normal voice. Sixty seconds is a very long time for you but may be barely enough for them to process your question.
- Pause often to let the Person catch up.

Maintain continuity. The Person's brain can only process one thought at a time. It will either ignore additional thoughts or stop processing. If it stops, it must start over from the beginning.

- Offer one thought. Wait and allow for processing and a response before offering another thought.

Doris: "I like your red coat."

Larry: (long pause.) "Thank you." (Another long pause while he is obviously trying to think of more to say.) "I think Amy gave it to me."

Doris: "She has good taste."

Doris waited until she was sure Larry was completely through talking before she said anything more. Even though Amy is their daughter, Doris didn't allude to that because that would have required Larry to make another connection--and take more time.

Larry: (Long pause.) "Thank you." (Smiles.)

Doris: "I like your hat too."

Doris finished one subject before she started another.

Avoid compound sentences that require the Person to consider two different issues.

Once, even before we knew anything was wrong, Bill and I took my dad out to dinner. I asked Bill if I could have his butter if he didn't want it. When he just sat there looking at his plate, I shrugged mentally and went on visiting with my dad. Five minutes later, Bill picked up his butter and put it on my plate. Years later, after Bill's diagnosis, I remembered that and understood that he'd been processing my question that whole time. — Marla (excerpt from Managing Cognitive Issues in Parkinson's and Other Lewy Body Disorders)

Marla's request required Bill to consider a) did he want the butter and b) could she have it. His LBD was early and so he was able to process both requests, but it took a long time.

- Avoid interrupting or trying to finish their sentences. The Person has to stop processing to consider your suggestion.

- When you must talk about two different things, say whatever you want the Person to focus on first so that they don't miss it. "Put on your coat and we can go for a ride" not "We can go for a ride after you put on your coat."

Use clarity. The Person's brain stumbles over complicated words, can't make clarifying guesses and may not be able to process concepts at all.

- Talk slowly and clearly. The Person can't use abstract thinking to clarify slurred or unclear words. Pause often to let the Person catch up. When a Person doesn't understand you, repeat your words or better yet, use different words.

- Use concrete terms. Talk about what you can see, hear and feel. Avoid compound words or abstract terms.

- Use object names of pronouns. "Is this glass yours?" rather than "Is this yours?" Figuring out what a pronoun refers to adds a level of processing. It also requires being able to do sequences and/or remembering past information.

- Avoid negative qualifiers. The Person's brain may skip over words like "not" and "never" that change the

190

meaning of a statement. "I'm staying here," works much better than "I'm not leaving" which the Person may hear as "I'm leaving." "I'll never stop loving you" may mean "I've stopped loving you." Simply say "I love you."

Stay in the moment. Time is a lost art for the Person.

Yesterday morning, the aide told Mom that I was coming this afternoon. By the time I got here, Mom was in a dither. She was afraid she'd missed me. -- Shirley.

Mrs. Bloom has no sense of time. Waiting a few hours, let alone a whole day, causes her to feel as though she has been waiting for something long overdue--and possibly missed.

- Wait until just before an event occurs to announce it: "I'm here to take you shopping." vs "I'll be there to take you shopping tomorrow." Or "Dinner is ready" vs "Dinner will be in an hour."

- Give the Person a task to complete while waiting. "Finish folding these clothes and then we can go" rather than "We can go in an hour." Their focus on this busy work will allow them to wait while staying in the moment.

You can no longer use what's happened in the past to justify what's happening in the present moment.

When Gerry accused me of lying about meeting my lover, I told him I'd never lied to him before and I wasn't about to start now. He just kept accusing me. -- Olivia

Olivia based her denial on the past, which is not accessible to Gerry. All he knows about is now, where his brain has told him that Olivia is being unfaithful and is planning to leave him. That irrevocable knowledge was painful enough, but now she has compounded her sins by lying about it. He is devastated. Since past history doesn't count anymore, Olivia

191

must address Gerry's present feelings of betrayal. Anything else will only increase his distress.

- Address accusations in the present by responding in an empathetic manner to the Person's present feelings.

Use acceptance. It is natural to want to interrupt a Person with a guessed word, to make a correction or to defend.

- If like Olivia, you want to defend, remind yourself that it will do no good. Olivia needs to accept Gerry's accusation as his truth and respond to his negative feelings instead.

- If you understand what the Person means, avoid correcting. If you know they are talking about the yellow house but they call it the yellow barn, let it go.

- If you need clarification, wait for a break in their talking or behavior. Then, ask simple questions to verify your guess, "Do you mean that (whatever your guess or correction is)?" or "Is this where you hurt (gently touch area)?

Respond to the negative feeling. It is fairly easy to respond to feelings that are positive. However, negative feelings are the ones that initiate unwanted behaviors. The longer a situation lasts, the stronger these already strong emotions become. The lasting-strength of a memory depends on the strength of its attached emotions. Therefore, it is important for their comfort and yours that you defuse the situation quickly.

When a Person accuses you, their negative emotions are in charge. It is important that you respond in a way that doesn't make the situation worse:

- Arguing increases the Person's anger.
- Explanations make them feel patronized and frustrated.
- Defending makes you sound like a liar to them.

On the other hand, validating negative feelings allows the Person to feel heard and thus, calmer. Once the negative feelings are gone or at least, less powerful, you can use distraction to move on to something more pleasant.

Align with the feeling. If the Person is out of control, aligning with the feeling may be the only way you will be able to connect initially. Follow the steps in Chapter 19-Working with Present Abilities. Briefly:

- Express similar, but less intense feelings towards the same "enemy."
- Use soft crooning to help the person feel rescued and safe with you.
- Deep breathe and let them join you.
- When they are calm, word your plans to solve the problem as an invitation for them to participate.

Apologize. When a Person feels wronged and voices an accusation, their concern needs to recognized and validated so that the negative feeling will vanish. This often means apologizing for something you didn't do.

The last time Gerry accused me of infidelity, I just told him I was sorry. I was amazed. Once I'd accepted his way of seeing things, he calmed right down. Then, when I suggested we go have lunch, he was happy to go. - Olivia

Olivia's apology defused the situation. Gerry felt heard and was able to let go of his painful negative feelings and relax so that Olivia was then able to use his short attention span to deflect his attention onto something more pleasant.

Apologizing for something you didn't do can be very difficult. But the bottom line is that you can't change the Person's reality. You can change YOUR response and that can then change the Person's whole demeanor. Saying "I'm sorry" validates the Person's complaint, defuses their anger and allows you both to move on.

When you apologize, be sincere even if you didn't do anything wrong. Without sincerity, your apology may not work. You can justify to yourself an "I'm sorry" statement about something you didn't do by:

- Thinking about how sorry you are that the Person is having to experience this unhappy experience, even though it is not your reality.
- Considering yourself an improv actor in the Person's drama.
- Accepting apologizing as a tool that defuses the Person's negative feelings before they result in greater decreases of their comfort level.

Don't worry that your apology will cause the Person to believe even more firmly in their accusation. First, they already believe as firmly as they possibly can. Even if they didn't, developing a stronger belief requires the ability to make judgments--abstract thinking.

Instead, focus on trying to limit their memory of the event. The sooner you defuse a situation, the weaker the negative emotions will be and thus, the less likelihood that they will be remembered.

Divert or distract. Once the Person is calm enough to respond normally, use distraction to move them on to something else. Done quickly, this will likely dissipate any leftover negative feelings along with the memory of the event.

I learned the hard way that although distraction works well, I have to be sure Gerry can hear me first. If his own negative

194

feelings are "louder" than my words in his brain, I might as well save my breath. And so I have to do whatever I think will work best to calm him down. Sometimes that means apologizing. Sometimes, I show a little anger at whatever he is upset about and empathize with him. It just depends on the situation. But then, when he is calm enough to hear me I can suggest something like fixing him a dish of ice cream. He always goes for that! -- Olivia

Avoid criticism. The person with a normal brain hears a criticism and then uses abstract thinking to accept or reject it. Even so, it still takes many positives to overcome one negative criticism. The Person takes criticisms literally, just like they do compliments--and then they are stuck with it-- and the resulting negative feelings.

- Be careful to word comments and observations positively.

Working with Carol has really made me think about what I say and how often I word things negatively. Since she can no longer guess what I mean she takes everything at face value and responds negatively, which can lead to problems. I've learned to stop and think of a way to rephrase what I say so that it helps her instead of hurting her. For example, the other day she wanted to wear a blouse that was way too dressy. Instead of telling her that, I told her how lovely I thought she'd look in a more appropriate blouse. She accepted my judgment and we were both happy! -- Harold.

***

Responsive Care Takeaways for Being Engaging:

- Mindful listening requires your full attention and an understanding of what to listen for.

  Attitudes:

  - Empathy to help you better understand and accept what the Person is feeling and their reality.
  - Calm acceptance that provides a model the Person can mirror to help them let go of their own negative emotions.

  Actions:

  - Look for the nonverbal and emotional cues that become more likely--and more accurate--as language skills fade.
  - Be alert for underlying residual emotions that can trigger otherwise irrational behaviors.
  - Be alert for cues such as limping or cradling a possibly sore area. These may indicate irritants or illnesses which can draw the Person's focus and limit their ability to verbalize.

- Mindful listening allows you to hear what the Person can't communicate verbally.

Attitudes:

- Empathy, patience, simplicity, clarity and staying in the moment.
- Being cheerful, patient, relaxed and accepting.

- Responding to a Person in ways they can hear and understand greatly improves communication.

Actions:

- o Take your time, talk slowly, pause often and talk about only one subject at a time.

- o Enunciate clearly and repeat if necessary or use different words. Avoid pronouns and negative modifiers.

- o Avoid early warnings of coming events.

- o Avoid defenses that require past memory.

- o Avoid interruptions, corrections or defending. Use questions for clarifications rather than a statement.

- • ***Negative emotions block communication. The longer they last, the more they block.***

  Actions:

  - o Validate negative feelings instead of arguing, explaining or defending.

  - o If necessary, align with the feeling to show you are on their side.

- • Sincere apologies defuse angry accusations so that distractions can move the Person away from negative emotions.

  Attitude:

  - o Be sincere. Insincere apologies or compliments will be rejected.

  Action:

  - o Make copious use of apologies.

  Self-care:

  - o Let go of your normal resistance to apologizing for something you didn't do.

22. Keeping Track

A journal is a care partner's friend. With dementia's continual changes, an ongoing record of the journey can be very helpful. Symptoms and behaviors can seem random and uncontrollable. A journal helps you to find patterns and triggers.

It helps you to identify therapies that improve the situation over time and those that don't. It helps you to see changes that happen so gradually over time that they are easily missed by anyone who lives with them every day.

You can review the Person's past progress, with a record of the changes, behaviors, medications, techniques and alternative remedies used, reactions to each and anything else of importance. And finally, it is a safe place to vent.

I've found that there are a lot more things that I need to keep track of than I can possibly remember without help. I'm not a writer and I don't try to tell stories or anything like that. I don't even write in sentences very much. I mostly just jot down lists with dates and such. Then I have facts to support what I tell the doctor about Gerry's behavior and what I've done. It helps me too because I can see over time what worked and what didn't. -- Olivia

You don't have to write in your journal every day. It doesn't even have to be a journal. Some care partners even use a calendar.

Whatever you use, make it a habit to jot down anything about the Person's care, medications or activities that might have been involved with a behavioral episode, including:

- Triggers, patterns, times of day

- What you did to deflect the behavior and how it worked
- Medication or alternative options used
- Additional or new behaviors, including anything that might have triggered them

Evaluating your efforts. Once you've found a trigger and made an attempt to change the situation, take time to evaluate. This way you will have a better idea of how to prevent or decrease that particular stress in the future.

In your journal, keep a record of your efforts. Answer questions like these:

How did you know there was stress? Was there a certain behavior or action? What was the behavior's hidden message?

What was the stressor? How would you recognize it next time? What can you do to keep it from appearing again?

What did you do to change the situation? How effective were your efforts? What would you do differently next time?

Documenting concerns. Documenting information about any concerns you have gives you a record for comparison if the problem occurs again, and it helps you when it is time for a doctor's visit. Jot down such things as:

- Changes as they occur, as in sleeping or eating behavior, even small ones.
- Falls, with bruises or other damage along with the probable cause.
- Pain, along with its probable cause and what you've done to treat it.
- Existing illnesses such as diabetes or heart problems, medications and other treatments and how they work.

- Behavior that is new or unusual, even if it isn't disruptive.

A doctor or therapist needs to know:

- How often a behavior occurs and its severity.
- Is there a trigger, a pattern or a special time of day when the behavior is more likely?
- Medications taken prior to and/or after the event.
- What has worked in the past in a similar situation.
- What you've tried this time and how it worked.

When something bothers you, write it down. Then you'll have a record of exactly what happened. Doctor's visits are usually stressful. Without a written record, it is easy to forget the whole item or important parts of it.

Documenting your successes. When you solve a problem or find a new way to deal with a behavior, write it down. You'll have it for next time. Besides, writing down your successes as a great self-esteem booster!

Reducing stress. A journal is good self-care in that its use can reduce stress:

- It provides accurate reports. You have a record of necessary information available for family and medical personnel, or even yourself, written when it was fresh in your memory.
- It can be a reminder of good times. Document successes and happy memories too. Then when you have a bad day, you have something to go back to and see that it can be better.
- It can be a place to vent, where your negative feelings won't hurt anyone. Once expressed and validated, your negative feelings will likely diminish, allowing you to

go back to your job as care partner with a more positive attitude.

***

Responsive Care Takeaways for Keeping Track:

- Journaling provides an ongoing record of the Person's progress, behaviors, the care partner's efforts at dealing with these and the results thereof.

  ### *Actions:*
  - o Record behaviors or any changes along with possible triggers and treatment.
  - o Take your journal with you to the Person's doctor appointments.
  - o Record your concerns so that you will have a record if it becomes a recurring problem.

  Self-care: Use journaling to assist your memory, remember good times and as a safe place to vent.

Section Four: Alternative Options

alternative options: *Non-drug remedies and interventions, that can be used alone or in combination with drug therapy.*

***

A variety of authorities from around the world agree that in most cases alternative options should be considered for behavior management before drugs.

Non-drug treatments should be used before medication is prescribed - unless the person with dementia or others are at risk of severe harm. -- Alzheimer's Association.

People with dementia who develop non-cognitive symptoms or behaviors that challenge should be offered a drug in the first instance only if they are severely distressed or there is an immediate risk of harm to the person or others. -- Alzheimer's Australia

Because available drugs used to treat behaviors have modest efficacy at best, are associated with notable risks, and do not address behaviors most distressing for families, non-drug options are recommended as first-line treatments or if necessary, in parallel with drug or other treatment options. -- Gitlin, et al.[30]

***

Alternative options include a multitude of alternative therapies and interventions that help you to prevent, limit or manage behaviors with fewer drugs while increasing quality of life for both care partner and Person. They are limited only by your imagination. The suggestions in this book are just a start. As you become used to thinking outside the (pill)box, you will come up with others. Alternative options can be divided into several categories. Some are initially preventive but continue to be helpful even after dementia appears.

- **Rehabilitation therapies,** procedures that the medical community has used for years to limit, adapt to, or regenerate waning physical abilities, thus providing the Person with a better quality of life.

- **Healthy living practices,** routines that give the body better resources to do the best it can with what it has.

- **Preventive measures,** techniques that prevent problems before they happen by "dementia-proofing" the environment and being alert for physical discomfort.

- **Relaxation exercises,** therapies and techniques that directly counteract the effects of stress by slowing the breathing rate, relaxing muscles and lowering blood pressure.

- **Engagement skills,** techniques used to interact with the Person in ways that preserve personhood, respect and keep communication open.

- **Alternative therapies**, those that use a sense pathway to increase the feel-good chemicals in the body that foster positive feelings.

- **Enhancing activities,** which also stimulate the feel-good chemicals in the body and generate positive feelings.

- **Sports, hobbies and special interests,** activities that combine at least two of the above categories while adding feelings of accomplishment and normality.

23. Rehabilitative Therapies

Physical therapy, occupational therapy and speech therapy have been in dementia treatment plans for years. Psychological therapy or counseling is also a valuable tool. These therapies all decrease behaviors by helping the Person to adapt to changes and make the most of life as it is. This includes identifying and using remaining strengths and abilities. The therapist helps you and your Person find ways to use these strengths to minimize the inevitable losses that dementia brings.

Physical Therapy

Physical therapy (PT) helps a Person use remaining physical abilities and strengths to improve muscles, balance and mobility, manage pain and prevent falls.[31]

Improving muscle strength, balance and mobility: While the elderly and any Person are all at risk, these problems are more serious with LBD or PD. Improving or even maintaining balance, muscle strength and/or mobility will prevent falls and related pain. Equally important, it improves one's sense of self-worth.

Managing pain: While dementia seldom causes pain, it is often present due to age and age-related disorders such as arthritis. Most pain drugs are on the at-risk-for-sensitivity list and should be avoided. PT often includes ongoing exercises that strengthen muscles and replace or reduce the need for pain medication.

Earl gets really ornery when he hurts. At first, I didn't understand why. But then I realized that he was always better after his PT session. I asked the therapist and she told me that his muscles probably hurt less when he moved them. Wow! I thought the PT was just to keep him mobile...a good enough reason to go all by itself, but now I know that it also keeps Earl from hurting as much. – Wanda

Our bodies are made to move. Physical therapy helps the person who hasn't been moving enough to stretch their muscles and keep them from cramping up.

Occupational Therapy

The occupational therapist[32] focuses on daily living skills, helping the Person to adapt and compensate for lost skills and to maintain feelings of usefulness and self-worth.

Maintaining strengths: The therapist helps your Person identify existing skills and strengths that can be used to compensate for lost skills. The goal is for them to do as much self-care, be as independent and feel as useful as possible.

Maintaining self-worth: The therapist guides in the choosing of meaningful activities and tasks while maintaining safety. The goal is for the Person to feel useful and actively invested in something that holds their interest.

Speech Therapy

The speech therapist focuses on throat functions: verbal communication and swallowing.

Communication: Parkinson's and Lewy body dementia often causes soft speech to be an issue. Programs like LSVT Big and Loud[©] [33] program, where people are taught to exaggerate their speech, can make a difference.

Mason's voice is getting very low and weak, and he shuffles a lot. These symptoms aren't surprising, but they are annoying. We joined a Big and Loud[©] group. I go too. That way, I can help him with his exercises at home. I didn't expect it to be such fun, but it really is. I'm so glad we are going. -- Iris

Swallowing: Dementia often affects a Person's ability to swallow. The therapist teaches ways to improve your Person's ability to swallow and ways to compensate for this issue, such as using thickened fluids.

Psychological Therapy

There is a stigma attached to needing help dealing with emotions. Therefore, psychological therapy, where a professional counselor helps their clients to deal with emotional issues is less likely to be recommended by physicians or considered by care partners. It is usually easier to accept the need for medical help than it is to accept that we might benefit from psychological guidance.

Don't let this stop you. Dementia care brings about a multitude of emotions, many of them negative. Just as good medical advice helps one to deal with physical problems, good psychological advice can help sort out and deal with these emotions.

"John said that our psychologist...contributed in some ways as much to his feeling of well-being as did his neurologist and the medicines he prescribed." -- Pat Snyder in her book, Treasures in the Darkness.[34]

Counseling can help individuals, couples and families work out the changes, stresses, grief and disruptions related to dementia.

Change: Dementias come with continual changes. You and anyone involved with your Person must change too. The counseling session is a great place to discuss this process.

Stress: Dementia is emotionally stressful for everyone in so many ways. Part of a counselor's job is to know a variety of ways to deal with stress.

When my sister went on hospice, I moved to her home and became her care partner. I was in a strange city where I had no friends. The hospice social worker took me walking with her. It was great. I was able to vent and talk about my own issues instead of focusing on my sister's--and I got some exercise. I returned as a much better caregiver to my sister. – Bonnie, sister of Lucy

Social workers can provide good counseling too, as they did for Bonnie.

Grief: Any progressively degenerative disease causes continual losses to be grieved as you go. As a Person loses one ability after the other, grief will follow, for both the Person and for the care partner who must pick up the slack.

- *Action:* Be sure to choose a counselor who is familiar with ambiguous, ongoing grief as well as the basic grief process that includes shock, depression, anger, bargaining and acceptance.

Carter's personality is fading away before my eyes. Oh, I still love him, but it's different now. He is no longer the man I can go to with my problems or often even my joys. I find that I am grieving the loss of the man I used to know. -- Gwen

Anticipatory grief like Gwen's is almost always going to be part of the care partner's journey. Families must deal with two deaths, the slow fading of a loved one's personality well before the actual physical death.

Family disagreements: Especially in blended families, various members of the family may not support the care partner, or may not believe the seriousness of the situation.

208

- *Action:* Family counseling may bring separate factions together or may help you to accept and move on.

***

Responsive Care Takeaways for Rehabilitative Therapies:

- Physical, occupational and speech therapy helps to use remaining skills, manage pain, maintain independence and improve self-worth.
- Psychological counseling helps the Person, care partners and other family members deal with the dementia-related changes.

    Attitude: Accept the need for psychological help as being as needed and useful as medical help.

    Actions:

    Seek help for such issues as dementia-related relationship issues, stress, grief or family disagreements.

    Use counseling to assist in decreasing your normal resistance to change and make this hard job a little easier.

    Pay attention to a counselor's suggestions about ways to deal with stress.

    Be sure to choose a counselor well-versed in grief counseling, including that specific to dementia.

    Self-care: Make sure you address your own physical, occupational and psychological issues as well as the Person's.

24. Preventive Measures

Preventive measures are those that you use to predict and then remove or decrease triggers of unwanted behavior. Save yourself and your Person unnecessary anguish, pain and distress by being alert for possible issues. Think about what these triggers might be and then consider how you can make the necessary changes. In improv, this is "setting the stage." Three things to consider are environmental control, infection control and pain management.

Environmental Control

Dementia makes it stressful to deal with change, variety or extremes. With added stress, behaviors often follow. However, you can do a lot to change the Person's external environment, even before any of these symptoms appear. Here are some triggers and suggested actions:

Extremes. A Person has difficulty focusing on more than one thing at a time. Too much of anything can cause confusion, which will often be expressed as agitation and irritation.

> ***Action:*** Eliminate clutter. Clear off counters, dresser and table tops, put away magazines, remove small area rugs.

Mom likes to have her own things around her. They help her to stay more alert in the care facility where she lives. But I've learned to put out only a few at a time. Too many and she gets agitated. – Shirley

With only a few personal items around her, Shirley's mom can relax and enjoy each one. Shirley can change them occasionally so that her mom can enjoy more of her own things over time.

Crowds. Large groups of people cause the same problems that other extremes do. Crowds also have a normal bustle, with movement, noise and excitement, which adds to the confusion.

Actions:

- Limit visitors to one at a time when possible and never more than two or three.
- Avoid crowds. Learn when malls are least crowded and go shopping or walking then.
- ***A more creative action:*** Find a way to isolate the Person from the stressful hubbub of noisy active groups while still participating.

Donna has always loved the zoo. It's really crowded Saturdays but we decided to go anyway. I brought along her ear-buds and MP3 player, so she could "tune out" kids and noise with music when she needed to. We stopped to rest in quieter spots so she could take some time to listen to her music and regroup. After about 2 hours she was beat; losing focus and balance...that happens when she get tired...but the ear buds and quieter places worked. She had a great time.[35] – *Nick*

Donna's MP3 player allowed her to spend an afternoon doing something she loved, even in a crowded atmosphere. Adaptation is the name of the game!

Sensitivities: Many caregivers report that their loved ones perceive light as much brighter than it actually is. Likewise, noise may appear not only louder but distorted as well, adding fear.

- *Action:* Avoid bright lights and loud noises.
- ***A more creative action:*** Use sunshades and sunglasses outdoors and even indoors if the light feels too intense.

Media, especially the TV: As the ability to differentiate between fact and fiction decreases, the Person can perceive an exciting or scary television show as real and thus find it very stressful.

> *Action:* Monitor the TV and make an effort to choose shows less likely to cause stress. Choose shows without a plot—sports, game or travel shows.

> *A more creative action:* Provide some low-stress DVDs for the Person to choose from instead of TV programs. This helps to maintain a sense of control while limiting opportunities for stress.

Change. With a limited ability to adapt and learn, Persons living with dementia feel more in control of their lives with repetition than variety and with familiarity instead of newness.

I used to be a risk-taker, an "adrenalin junkie," seeking out thrills to fulfill my need for excitement. Now my disorder provides all the challenges I need.[36] — Charles Schneider

Change-generated feelings of insecurity and discomfort are likely to be expressed with unwanted behaviors.

Actions:

- *Develop routines and rituals* for bedtime, eating, traveling or any common activity. They have a soothing, almost mesmerizing quality. When the Person knows exactly what to expect, it is easier to take that next step, and the next.

- *Keep home feeling safe.* Home is the most familiar place and feels the safest. Maintain that by avoiding any changes in appearance or location of furniture and furnishings.

- *Take familiar outings.* Choose the same destinations, take the same routes, ask for the same table, go through the aisles in the same sequence, etc.

- *Add familiar objects.* Personal items such as photos on the dresser of an assisted living space or a favorite blanket while traveling can make the difference between comfort and anxiety.

- *Buy the same clothes.* Don't even change the color. The comfort of familiarity is much more important than style.

- *Limit needed changes.* Even when changes are needed for better functioning, make them minimal. For example, Velcro-fastened shoes foster independence, but choose the same color and style as the Person's old lace-up shoes.

  - *Use cues.* A specific routine or article can signal the advent of a regular event.

Tony knows that when I put a lap blanket over his knees it's time for a nap and when I ask him to set the table, he knows that it is time to eat. -- Angela

  - *Use timers to set limits.* This helps your Person to move past their "in the now" orientation. "I will be back before the timer rings" helps them to wait more easily.

Tony doesn't follow me into the bathroom since I started using a timer. He just watches the timer instead. -- Angela

  - For more suggestions, review the fact sheet about Environmental Adaptations to Dementia[37] offered by the Canadian Psychological Assn.

Infection Control

Because Lewy bodies can compromise the immune system, infections are especially common with this type of dementia. However, as any dementia progresses, the immune system becomes less effective. An increase in behaviors or other dementia symptoms can be the first sign of an infection. Urinary tract infections are the most common, but so is pneumonia, as well as skin and GI tract infections.

Do not ignore symptoms of a possible infection. These vary with the type of infection, but include:

- fever over 101 degrees, chills
- swollen red areas
- obviously infected areas
- nausea
- abdominal pain
- a sudden increase in behaviors or other dementia symptoms.

To prevent infections, make sure the Person:

- drinks plenty of water
- uses good personal hygiene
- avoids choking
- avoids pressure sores
- doesn't have any unusual skin itching, lesions or pain

Once an infection is present it should be addressed medically. The doctor's plan of treatment will depend on the type of infection.

Pain Management

With age, arthritis and other painful illnesses become common. Pain decreases comfort and increases stress. Both lead to behaviors. The first step to decreasing pain is often to determine that it is present at all; that the reason for behaviors such as irritability is due to pain and not something else.

When Carol gets agitated, I suspect she is hurting somewhere. I know she's susceptible to UTIs but that she also has occasional digestive issues that can be painful. It's like being a detective. I just make some guesses and ask some questions. -- Harold

Harold uses his knowledge of Carol to identify pain as her probable stressor, rather than something in the environment or emotional stress. Next, he needs to find out what is causing the pain.

Identifying the pain. Carol may not be able to communicate about her pain accurately.

Issue: A Person may have difficulty connecting their "bad" feeling with a cause or perhaps, even a place on their body.

> ***Action:*** Use gentle questions and pointing to parts of the body.

Issue: A Person with impaired language skills may say the wrong word or none at all.

Sometimes Carol can tell me what is wrong but she often uses the wrong words. She might say her elbow hurts when it is really her knee. Once she told me her stomach hurt but what was really wrong was that she had a UTI and her urinary tract was irritated and burning. I've learned to pay more attention to where she puts her hands than what she says. -- Harold

> ***Action:*** Watch the gestures and ask for more information.

Issue: The pain may be delusional--real only to the Person. Nevertheless, it can be every bit as painful as if it were real.

Gerry complains a lot about aches and pains that neither I nor the doctor can find a reason for. At first I just told him to ignore them and they'd go away but of course, they didn't. Then I got smart and realized that I should treat this "false" pain was like any other delusion. I told him I was so sorry he hurt, gave him a Tums and told him that it would fix the pain. It did--and it gave him an extra boost of calcium at the same time! -- Olivia

216

Action: Consider placebos, either something safe for the Person like Tums (Check with the doctor to be sure!), or a prescription from the doctor.

Treating the pain: Most pain drugs are more likely than not to be problematic. Try these first:

- *Empathy* (Chapter 20), acceptance (Chapter 18) and communication skills (Chapter 21) to identify the issue, comfort and distract.

- *Alternative therapies* (Chapter 27) such as touch and massage to soothe and relax.

- *Enhancing activities* (Chapter 28) such as music and humor to distract and calm.

- *Rehabilitation therapy* (Chapter 23) to improve movement and strength and provide alternative ways of doing presently painful tasks.

If alternative options aren't enough, consider:

- Acetaminophen (Tylenol) is usually safe in small doses for short periods of times, but should be given only with a doctor's knowledge.

- Avoid over-the-counter drugs like Advil and Aleve that have side effects that can affect the GI tract and heart.

- Avoid using strong narcotics, antipsychotics, anti-anxiety drugs or other drugs known to be dementia-sensitive to treat pain. The side effects can be worse than the pain.

- If the doctor prescribes a mild narcotic, use it sparingly and with careful monitoring. All narcotics tend to be constipating and even the milder ones may be dementia-sensitive.

- If medical marijuana is legal in your state, talk to the supplier about one that treats pain without causing psychedelic events. It can often provide good pain relief with few side effects. However, it may be costly and is seldom covered by insurance.

Try these drugs combined with alternative options before opting to use them alone. The results are usually better, and require smaller doses than with a drug-only regime.

***

Responsive Care Takeaways for Preventive Measures:

- Taking steps to predict and remove triggers related to the environment, infections and pain saves unnecessary distress.

    Attitude: A willingness and patience for finding and dealing with the problem instead of using drugs as a quick fix.

    Actions:

    Monitor your environment to eliminate confusing, over-stimulating or distracting events. Maintain continuity with practices such as routines, cues for transitions and the presence of familiar objects.

    Use infection prevention measures such as ensuring adequate fluids regularly. Respond to symptoms of an infection quickly, usually with medical care rather than home remedies.

- A Person may use behaviors to express pain that they can't recognize or explain.

    Action: Use gentle questions and touch, watch for gestures. Treat with empathy, alternate therapies and distractions before resorting to drugs and then use the mildest, safest drugs possible.

25. Healthy Living Practices

Healthy living practices are also preventive measures. They provide the resources the body and brain uses to maintain general health, fight disease, deal with stress and reduce behaviors. They decrease the risk of most illnesses including dementia. Even after dementia is present, these practices provide fuel and free up internal resources, enabling it to better deal with dementia-related damage. As people age and bodies must work harder to maintain status quo, these practices become even more important.

Exercise

Many experts say that regular physical activity is more helpful with dementia than any drug. It helps to maintain a higher level of functioning for a longer time by:

- Increasing oxygen to the brain, thus providing more fuel for functions such as thinking and maintenance of the immune system.
- Increasing blood and oxygen to the muscles, which strengthens them and improves balance and grip strength.
- Releasing "feel good" hormones, thus decreasing depression.[38]
- Adding sociability when exercising is done with other people.
- Greatly increasing quality of life, due to all of the above.

Physical exercise comes in many forms. It can be done:

- In a rehab setting at a physical therapy clinic.
- In a group, as with a Big and Loud© class.

- In water, as with a water aerobics class or swimming laps.
- At home, using a video as a guide or with the care partner.
- Outside or in a mall, walking with a partner.
- As part of an activity, as with dancing or golf.

Requirements for best results are that exercise is:

- Challenging, but not painful.
- Enjoyable, so that the person will want to continue to do it.
- Regular. Daily is ideal; a half-hour three times a week is good; any amount helps.

Even the wheelchair-bound can exercise.

The facility where my mother spent her last years offered a regular exercise class for wheelchair-bound residents. Mom loved to go. They even played music and we "danced." I'd hold her hands and she'd move the wheelchair with her feet. Everyone had a good time and left feeling energized. – Edith, daughter of Myrtle

Active exercise, where a Person moves their own body is best as my mom did, but even passive exercise is better than none. As a nurse, I've provided passive exercise by moving limbs of patients who couldn't do it themselves. However, you don't have to be a nurse to do this. Just bend and straighten each of the Person's limbs at elbows and knees five to ten times, several times a day.

Hydration

The body is over 50% water. Water keeps cells, tissues and organs in good condition, transports nutrients, prevents constipation and regulates temperature. A Person needs more fluids if they are on diuretics, drinking coffee or alcohol, in dry humidity or if they are losing fluids through fever, sweating, vomiting or diarrhea.

Dehydration symptoms include fatigue, constipation, headaches, nausea, muscle cramps, confusion and behaviors. If your Person:

Forgets to drink. Keep a glass of water nearby, but don't expect your Person to remember to drink even then. Offer a drink every hour or so.

Refuses to drink to avoid the bother of toileting. If reasoning is still present, explain that adequate water intake makes the kidneys function better and actually decreases trips to the bathroom.

Nathan resisted drinking because "It will just come right out again." I tried to tell him that it was actually the opposite and he'd be in the bathroom less often but that didn't make any sense to him. Then I remembered that he always orders lemon-flavored water in restaurants and so I tried that. It worked! Now we drink lots of "restaurant water." -- Elsie

Adding a favorite flavor to water as Elsie did will likely work better with the Person whose dementia has advanced past the ability to reason very much. Offering it at regular intervals will turn it into an expected ritual and make it more acceptable too. Also, Elsie drank with Nathan. That can help too. Besides, care partners need adequate fluids just as much as their loved ones do.

Is afraid to drink, due to swallowing issues. Thickened fluids are easier to swallow. A speech therapist can teach ways of drinking that are less likely to cause choking.

Sleep

Sleep is the time when the body actively restores and strengthens its resources. An elderly or infirm person needs about 7 to 9 hours of sleep a night to function properly. The symptoms from lack of adequate sleep include: confusion and behaviors, less muscle strength, decreased function of vital organs, pain sensitivity, diabetes risks and a weak immune system.

Sleep problems are common with all dementias and can start early for those who experience Active Dreams (RBD). Breathing problems, chronic pain from arthritis, an upset stomach, mood problems or an overactive bladder can also interfere with sleep.

In Chapter 13-Being Flexible, Rhonda talks about how Steve watched a detective story on TV and then had active dreams at night. After identifying the problem, she found a more calming program for him to watch. Dealing with other reasons for poor sleeping is similar: Once you've identified the problem, find a remedy. Often it will be in the list below:

- Regular sleep and wake schedule.
- A relaxing and unexciting bedtime routine.
- Avoid exciting media programs at any time of the day and exciting visitors within 2-3 hours of bedtime.
- A dark, quiet and cool room used only for sleeping.
- Avoid caffeine or alcohol within 2-3 hours of bedtime.
- Avoid nicotine, a stimulant that can cause insomnia.
- Avoid sleeping aids; they tend to be dementia-sensitive.
- Melatonin (a natural hormone), in small doses an hour before bedtime may help. Do not use in the middle of the night.

If the cause of sleeplessness is a dementia-related symptom such as Active Dreams, dementia drugs may help. They treat non-cognitive symptoms as well as cognitive ones. The doctor may also recommend one of the milder antipsychotics, such as Seroquel. Use this with extreme caution. It works wonders for some and causes others great distress.

If the cause of sleeplessness is pain, see pain management, in Chapter 24-Preventive Measures.

Diet

Experts know that a Mediterranean diet[39] can reduce the risk of dementia. It may also decrease already present cognitive symptoms. In addition, there is some evidence that it can improve dementia-compromised immune systems and blood circulation. Its antioxidants, vitamins, minerals and fibers work together to help protect against many other chronic diseases as well.

Foods in a Mediterranean diet include:

- Vegetables, fruits, beans, whole grains, nuts and a little wine.
- Proteins such as eggs, cheese, yogurt, fish, a little poultry, but very little red meat.
- Unsaturated fats such as extra virgin olive oil or canola oil.

Choose foods that are:

Fresh or quick frozen. These retain their nutritional value best. Quick frozen can actually be better than fresh because the foods are processed at their most optimum time.

Unprocessed. Processed food will often include less healthy substances such as white flour or corn syrup. Labels should show no more than two items besides the food itself. For instance, clam chowder can have two ingredients besides the clams, milk, spices and vegetables.

Raw, steamed or grilled. These do not remove nutrients as does boiling, or add saturated fats as does frying. Baking can also work as long as the oils from the meat drain away from the food.

Properly prepared foods decrease the risk of metabolic syndrome, a combination of high blood pressure, high blood sugar, unhealthy cholesterol levels and abdominal fat.

Nutrition

Nutrition refers to the specific nutrients that we need to have healthy bodies. With a few exceptions, nutrients from food are better than supplements. These are especially helpful:

Antioxidants (Vitamins A, D and E, and Coenzyme Q10) support a healthy immune system, freeing up body resources to deal with dementia symptoms and other stresses. **Warning:** These are fat-soluble. Any excess is stored rather than excreted. The large doses often recommended may therefore cause liver damage.

I still give Carol Vitamin D supplements and I take them too. Our doctor told me that it is difficult for the elderly or infirm to get enough of this vitamin naturally, even if they live in a sun belt. Since we live where it snows in the winter, I'm sure we don't get enough! -- Harold

Vitamin D is one of the few supplements that many doctors still recommend. Consult your doctor about the amount.

Water-Soluble Vitamins (Vitamins C, B6, B12, folic acid) support a healthy immune system and decrease stress. They are excreted in the urine. Food is still the best source, but supplements can usually be taken safely in normal doses.

Omega Fatty Acids help with digestion, decrease infections and improve blood pressure, all systems affected by LBD. Fish, especially salmon, is the best source. Nuts, dry beans, broccoli and winter squash also have these nutrients in lesser quantities. Coconut oil does too, but its value is conflicting because it is saturated, thus harder to metabolize.

***

Responsive Care Takeaways for Healthy Living Practices:

- Healthy living practices provide the body with resources to maintain health, fight disease and deal with stress

  Attitudes:
  - Persistence and determination about maintaining a healthy routine for you and the Person.
  - Resistance to slacking off and going back to old, often easier but less healthy routines.

- Regular physical activity may be more helpful with dementia than any drug.

  Action: Develop a regular routine for the Person that is lightly challenging and enjoyable.

- Dehydration symptoms include fatigue, constipation, headaches, nausea, muscle cramps, confusion and behaviors.

  Action: Assure adequate fluids by setting up a drinking schedule and using thickened fluids if needed.

- An elderly or infirm person needs 7 to 9 hours of sleep for restoring resources. Sleep deprivation symptoms: confusion, decreased organ function, pain sensitivity and poor immunity.

    Action: Set up a sleep routine that addresses the Person's specific issues and facilitates their sleep. Include things that foster sleep and avoid those that stimulate.

- The Mediterranean diet may decrease dementia symptoms, improve the immune system and blood circulation.

    Action: Adapt cooking styles to put more focus on the foods in the Mediterranean diet and the healthiest forms of food preparation.

- Proper nutrition gives the body the fuel it needs to function well. Except for a few cases, food provides better nutrition than supplements.

    Action: Work with the Person's health care team to assure that the Person gets adequate antioxidants, vitamins and omega fatty acids. Add Vitamin D supplements with the doctor's approval.

26. Relaxation Exercises

Relaxing the body relaxes the mind and lowers stress. The exercises can be very short, as with deep breathing or take much longer, as with guided relaxation. Practicing longer ones regularly makes it easier to do the quick ones when needed. A Person will likely need do them mirroring the care partner unless they've been doing an exercise prior to the onset of dementia.

Deep Breathing is a quick exercise that you can stop and do anytime life becomes stressful. It draws oxygen into the lungs and provides more fuel for the brain so that it can function better.

Deep breathing is one of the best relaxation exercises for the Person. It is contagious and so if you deep breathe, they will imitate you and you both will benefit!

Take three deep breaths and watch the Person deep breathe along with you.

I've learned to take a quick time out whenever I feel really stressed by something Nathan does and I can't get away. I just close my eyes and take about three deep breaths. Then I can usually get back to whatever we've been doing with more patience. It's funny, but I notice that Nathan is usually more calm then too. I guess he's been deep breathing right along with me -- Elsie

Meditation is the process of sitting quietly and clearing the mind. It can last a few minutes or as long as you like. Scientific trials have shown that meditation lowers stress and increases clarity of thought.[40] To do a simple meditation:

- Sit in a quiet place paying attention to nothing but your breathing.

- Let your mind go blank and feel yourself fall into a meditative calm.

- When your mind wanders, as it will, gently pull it back to your breathing.

- Allow yourself to continue this for as long as you feel comfortable doing so, but at least for 5 minutes, extending the time as you become more comfortable doing so.

The calmness you feel after meditating will last long after you return to your busy life. Although meditating seems very simple, it usually takes some practice to learn to calm those busy thoughts. For more direction, check out this reference.[41]

Like most caregivers, I don't get enough sleep but naps don't work for me. I wake feeling grouchy. Don calls me a grizzly bear! – Darlene

Normal sleep comes in cycles that last about ninety minutes each. A nap usually doesn't get further than the first portion of the cycle. When it does, the napper may wake up feeling grouchy due to an uncompleted cycle. Darlene might try meditating instead of napping. There are no "cycles" in meditation. A short session can be quite helpful and the longer it lasts, the more helpful it can be.

Yoga takes meditation a step further by adding exercise and deep breathing. Yoga may also help dementia patients and their care partners socialize and just plain feel better.[42] While yoga can be extreme, it can also be gentle and can even be done from a chair. However, it does take some training, thus may be better for the care partner than for the Person unless they start doing the exercises while abstract thinking is still intact.

I've done yoga for years. It is one of the things I do now for respite. One of the days that Gerry goes to day care, I take a yoga class. -- Olivia

Yoga can require more learning and many people do attend a weekly class as motivation. Such exercises are easier to continue doing in a group, although once you know some movements, you can do them at home for a quick pickup.

Guided relaxation is the process of following directions given in a soft, relaxing voice. It can take a variety of forms, from relaxing muscles to suggesting pleasant thoughts. It can last from 15 minutes to an hour. The Inner Health Studio[43] offers several different kinds of free guided relaxation experiences. Try several and find the one you, your loved one, or both like best.

Tai Chi is a low impact exercise that combines meditation, deep breathing and yoga, in a form easily practiced by seniors--and Persons. It is another exercise that is usually done in groups but can easily be done at home once you learn how.

Carol and I do Tai Chi every morning after breakfast. I got a DVD and we just follow the instructor. Carol loves it because it is so slow and she can easily keep up. -- Harold

***

Responsive Care Takeaways for Relaxation Exercises:

- Relaxation exercises relax the mind as well as the body. Most of them can be done in a modeling/ mirroring mode, where the Person follows someone else's lead.

    Attitude: Welcome relaxation exercises as useful for bringing back the calm focus lost while dealing with stressful events and for daily maintenance.

- Deep breathing is a quick and effective relaxation exercise you can use almost anywhere and as often as needed.

- Meditation is useful for relaxing and improves clarity long after a session is done. It does take time to learn to do correctly

- Yoga adds the advantages of exercise and deep breathing to meditation. Often done in a group, it adds sociability and peer motivation.

- With guided relaxation, you can both follow someone else's recorded or live directions.

- Tai Chi is a slow-moving, low-impact exercise that combines meditation, deep breathing and yoga.

    Actions:

    o Find a long relaxation exercise style you enjoy and do it regularly.

    o Use deep breathing in impromptu situations as needed.

    o Do relaxation exercises with the Person to relax both of you.

230

27. Using the Sense Pathways

essential oils: *Highly concentrated extracts from flowers, leaves, and other plant parts.*

diffuser: *a device that disperses essential oils into the surrounding air. Do not use a warm air humidifier as a diffuser. It heats the oils and makes them less effective.*

aromatherapy: *Using a diffuser to spread aromatic and healing essential oils into the air around the Person and anyone else in the area.*

Touch therapy: *Using one's hands to stimulate the tactile pathways to the brain. May or may not involve the use of essential oils.*

Sound therapy: *Using the sense of hearing as its pathway into the brain. Includes music, rhythm and vibration.*

Visual stimulation: *Uses light, color, shape and motion to stimulate and relax.*

**

In Chapter 3, The Senses, we discussed how the five senses travel to the brain via their own pathways. These pathways can also be used to decrease behaviors in a variety of ways. Most require some effort by the care partner or a professional but this is offset by the advantages such as a decreased need for drugs and a better quality of life.

The senses follow routes that pass close to the brain's emotional center. Sense-based therapies, also called "alternative therapies," are often used to alter negative feelings and foster positive ones. They can help to calm the anxious, relax the irritable, elevate the despondent and even clear up some of the fogginess at times. On the down side, the changes are seldom permanent. Like a pill that one must take regularly to work, these therapies must also be used regularly to be effective.

Each sense delivers information to the brain via a different pathway. If one doesn't work, you can try another or try using two pathways at once. An example of this is using smell and touch with massage.

Essential Oils

Many alternative therapies use essential oils, which are natural substances infused from plants that have a variety of helpful properties and few side effects. Essential oils are highly concentrated natural, usually aromatic, plant oils. Their side effects and sensitivity issues are usually fewer and when present, much milder than with manufactured drugs. These natural substances typically utilize senses such as smell to access the same areas of the brain that drugs do.

I keep a diffuser going during the day. It is such an easy way to soothe and calm Gerry--and it helps me too. -- Olivia

I use essential oils when I massage Carol's legs in the evening. The aromas soothe the mind as well as the muscles. -- Harold.

I diffuse some of the more invigorating oils when I want Carter to be more alert. -- Gwen

With dementia, these oils are mainly used for relaxation, easing depression, decreasing anxiety and insomnia and improving clarity.

There are a growing number of essential oil distributors, but not all are equal. There are several online sites that compare companies. You should look for:

- *Quality.* You want an oil that does the job it is supposed to do. Customer reviews can be helpful here.
- *Purity and testing practices.* The oils should be tested for purity regularly, preferably by an outside service.
- *Cost.* Prices vary greatly but the most expensive is not necessarily the best.

There are also a confusing number of essential oils available. Research the oils and their uses in books and online sites or ask your supplier which is best for your needs. These are the oils often used with dementia:[44]

- *Lavender:* Balancing strong emotions, insomnia.
- *Peppermint:* Stimulates the mind and calm nerves. As with any stimulant, best used in the morning.
- *Rosemary:* Similar to peppermint. Also may increase appetite and decrease constipation.
- *Bergamot:* Mood elevator used to relieve anxiety, agitation, mild depression and insomnia.
- *Lemon:* Used to calm and relax and to relieve anxiety and insomnia. May improve memory, digestion and immune system function.
- *Ylang ylang:* Eases depression, promotes sleep. Often combined with lemon oil.
- *Ginger:* Helps with digestion, loss of appetite and constipation.

Essential oils are administered in the following ways:

- *Inhaled:* Sniff the aromas directly from the bottle or a cloth or cotton ball soaked with the oil.
- *Diffused:* Use a cool-mist diffuser to distribute the aroma into a room. (Warning: Do not use a warm-air humidifier which can damage the oil.)
- *Sprayed:* Spray oil mixed with water onto linens or into a room.

- *Used with bathing:* Add a few drops to bathwater.
- *Used with massage:* Mix with a carrier oil such as almond or coconut and used as a massage lotion.
- *Ingested.* Use only those identified as "safe for internal use." Talk to your essential oil distributor about how to use these.

Oils should be used carefully just as drugs are. While on the whole, they are safer than drugs, they can also cause problems.

Start with the smallest amount recommended and increase slowly.

Mac got more agitated instead of calmer when I massaged him with some Lavender. I'm afraid to use it any more. -- Joanne

Joanne may have put too many drops of the essential oil in her massage oil. The oils listed above do not usually interact poorly with dementia. However, as with Mac, they can sometimes have an adverse (opposite) effect if too much is used at one time.

Pets. Be careful about using essential oils around pets, especially cats. The oils can often interfere with the animal's body processes. Keep pets out of the room when using a diffuser and avoid letting them lick you after a massage. Certain oils are more dangerous than others, but other considerations are also important, such as strength. For specifics, ask your essential oil dealer and your veterinarian.[45]

Aromatherapy

Depending on the oils involved, aromatherapy is used to calm or energize, to purify the air or to help the body fight bacteria, viruses and funguses. People living with Parkinson's and

LBD often lose their sense of smell early in their journey. This should not stop you from giving aromatherapy a try. Olfactory nerves (odor receptors) on the skin and throughout the body continue to work even when those in the nose may have failed.[46] Also, like most natural compounds, essential oils tend to have other active ingredients besides those that provide their distinctive smell. These continue to work.

Aromatherapy is easy to use without professional assistance and requires no effort on the Person's part. Just add oil, place it in a safe spot close to the Person and turn it on. Cost for the unit can be anywhere from about $15 to $120.

Most diffusers are cool-mist humidifiers. These have the added benefit of improving the humidity of a room, thus decreasing the amount of fluid the Person loses due to dry air. However, they do require monitoring since they stop when the water is gone.

The more expensive ones aren't humidifiers but they do have the advantage of needing less monitoring. They don't require water, have controls for the amount they diffuse and a timer that allows the unit to run in spaced intervals.

I set up a diffuser close to Mom's bed and used some oils recommended for inducing good sleep. She snuffles a lot at night and so I added an oil that facilitates breathing too. The diffuser is one of those that I can set to run off and on all night so that she gets the advantage of the oils for the whole night. I was afraid the motor would wake her up but it was quiet enough that it didn't. I think Mom sleeps better now. – Shirley

A cool-mist humidifier might have helped Shirley's mom's breathing even more, but that would have required monitoring which she wasn't available to do. Adding the oils to facilitate breathing was a compromise that apparently worked.

Touch Therapy

Non-custodial touch, massage, acupressure and acupuncture are all used to decrease anxiety, agitation, physical pain and stress while improving comfort, relaxation and reassurance.

A care partner can and should perform the simpler forms of this touch therapy although some types require training first. Others may require a professional whose services may or may not be covered by insurance.

Non-custodial touch is gentle touch, given voluntarily. Any gentle touch is beneficial, even that performed while helping with activities of daily living (ADLs). However, when it is given to show caring, the value increases exponentially.

I'm not a touchy person and Carol knew that. She also knew without a doubt that I loved her...as she did me. But now, just knowing isn't enough. She needs a lot more reassurance. -- Harold

With Carol's loss of abstract thinking, "just knowing" becomes impossible. She can no longer see tasks he does for love, like car care or doing the dishes, as signs of his caring. She needs ongoing direct evidence, like gentle touching.

Now I touch Carol every chance I get. When I go past her to get a drink of water, I rub her back a bit. When we are talking, I may just hold her hand. -- Harold

This simple but ever so valuable "therapy" is available to every care partner. All it takes is the willingness to use it.

I thought at first I might be going overboard and Carol would think something was fishy, but she just laps it up. -- Harold

Don't worry about overdoing it.

- All people initially react positively to pleasant touch, just the way they do to compliments (See Chapter 14- Being Positive). Then they use abstract reasoning to judge if the actions are sincere.
- Without abstract thinking, a Person accepts the touch at face value. Thus, the more attention you give them, the better it feels—and the better they feel.

I've seen a difference in her attitude. She's more positive and she doesn't get so agitated. -- Harold

Make your touch gentle but firm and move slowly.

- Touch that approaches too quickly or is too strong may feel threatening and initiate behaviors, or at the least, a startle reflex and just the opposite of what you intend.
- Touch that is too light may be ticklish and irritating and may cause the Person to draw back or even imagine that bugs are crawling on their skin.

Voluntary gentle touch conveys feelings such as care, concern and love. These feelings:

- Increase when mirrored back by the Person.
- Increase the Person's feelings of self-worth.
- Decrease negative feelings and behaviors.

Since I started making more effort to touch, Carol hasn't accused me of having another girlfriend. I guess she feels good enough about herself that she can accept that I'm here for her. -- Harold

- Can distract from a negative event, or provide direction by gently pulling the attention back to the job at hand.

I touch Carol gently when I want to pull her attention back to me. I give her a hug if she starts to get upset. It calms her down--if I do it soon enough. If I wait too long, she shrugs me off. The negative feelings have taken over and it is harder to get through to her. -- Harold

Massage therapy[47] soothes and relaxes. Professional therapists provide whole body massage and deep muscle massage. These can help with relaxation, relieve pain from tense muscles and decrease anxiety. With instruction, care partners can learn some helpful massage techniques to use at home. Make it a special time of togetherness between a care partner and Person.

Professional massage therapist can provide full body massages that can be wonderfully relaxing and stress reducing. Plan for weekly visits at the least for these to be their most effective.

Acupuncture[48] is an ancient Eastern art that involves the insertion and manipulation of needles in strategic points of the body by trained professionals. It can relieve pain and feelings such as anxiety and anger, in turn decreasing behaviors like combativeness. It can also improve sleep and speech. Like massage, acupuncture requires regular visits to be truly effective.

Acupressure[49] is similar to acupuncture, except that finger pressure is used instead of needles. It also provides the same type of help, except that since it is milder, it doesn't last as long. Care partners can learn to do at least parts of this therapy at home and care staff can learn to provide it in residential facilities.

I took a class and learned to give Mom hand and foot massages using essential oils. It would actually be worth it just because of the way she loves all the attention, but it does more. Mom has arthritis in her hands and I think it gives her more movement with less pain. I've shown some of the

238

residential staff what I've been doing and now they massage her hands too. -- Shirley

When touch therapies are performed by care partners, they have the added value of being a togetherness activity. The attention that Shirley's mom gets is likely of as much value as the pain relief.

Sound Therapy

Sound therapy uses the hearing pathway into the brain, thus it is processed in a different area than is language. Auditory stimulation improves mood, relaxation and cognition.

Music. Music involves more than hearing. The brain perceives music first as a sequence of basic sounds involving rhythm, timing, timbre and pitch. Next, the brain uses abstract thinking to identify these sounds as "musical" and the musical sequences as specific pieces of music. Then the information passes through a hub in the brain where it becomes associated closely with emotions and past memories. Because all of this occurs in an area of the brain where cognition is less likely to be damaged by dementia, these music-based skills often last long after language skills fade.[50]

In the Big and Loud© groups, there is a lot of singing. Persons normally unable to talk at all may be able to sing clearly and they may even be able to talk temporarily. Singing will usually improve any Person's ability to talk for up to several hours after a session ends.

I've noticed that after Carol attends a Big and Loud© group, she is much more alert for quite a while. She doesn't even shuffle as much! -- Harold

Rhythm is more basic. While it can be perceived as a basic aspect of sound, it can also be felt, as with one's heartbeat, or the internal jolts you experience as you listen to loud bass acoustics. This internal rhythm is used by the brain as a guide for movement, speaking and listening.[51]

The brain actually functions with internal rhythms of electrical (neuronal) energy. When something disrupts this, functioning becomes difficult. For example, with Parkinson's, walking turns to a shuffle. The beauty of rhythmic music is that it can temporarily reset the body's natural rhythms. The person with Parkinson's can walk better, or the Person living with dementia may be able to think more clearly. Playing a drum or other percussion instrument can also be uplifting and energizing.

At a recent conference, the last presentation of a very long day was one on the value of music and rhythm. The speaker got us all up on our feet and had us march around the room to a Sousa march. At first, I was resistant. I was tired just wanted to go home. But before long, I was caught up in the music and the camaraderie and was actually enjoying the activity. As we left the hall, James and I talked about how energized and spirited we both felt. -- Helen

Music and rhythm are also great for improving quality of life. Read more about this in Chapter 28-Enhancing Activities.

Other sound therapies. Sound therapists with special training use tuning forks to stimulate certain levels of vibration for increasing cognition, clarity and alertness. The vibrations seem to facilitate the parts of the brain to communicate better.[52]

A background of white noise can be soothing. A group in Australia had good results using a series of sessions with singing bowls to promote relaxation and inner well-being and relieve agitation.[53]

Physical therapists and chiropractors have used ultrasound, with vibrations too fast for the human ear to hear, for years to reduce local swelling, inflammation and pain. It is also used for imaging. Most pregnant woman have experienced ultrasound imaging of their fetus, but it could also be used with a Person with dementia to detect an internal growth.

Visual Stimulation

Vision, like hearing, uses its own pathway into the brain and is stored in a different place than is language. Therapy can utilize anything from artwork to movies to stimulate or relax.

Art and Mandalas: Any creative exercise, including art can be used as therapy. This is especially true if the person practiced any sort of art in the past, but is still valuable for any Person. It adds fun and purpose and increases one's sense of self-worth.

I got Dad some digestible paints. Last week when he was stressing over something, I asked him to paint some mandalas with me. It really did calm him down. I painted some too. It was fun and yes, I was calmer too by the time we finished. -- Ariel, daughter of Ralph

Drawing and coloring of mandalas, or sacred circles, is a special kind of art that uses the focus on concentric circles to promote concentration, relaxation and decrease stress, with the added bonus of the self-expression that any art provides.[54]

I try to meditate for a while every day. Starting out by tracing a mandala with my fingers helps me clear my mind. -- Ariel, daughter of Ralph

This is a good way to build concentration prior to meditating. Having a visual guide to follow helps but isn't necessary. You can trace an imaginary spiral on any flat surface with your finger and focus on making your circle gradually wider and wider or you can simply trace the infinity symbol over and over. Either one will help you clear your mind and relax it.

Passive activities such as watching a video or looking at a book or photo album can be entertaining but can also stimulate memories and emotions. Take care to choose content that will stimulate only positive emotions.

***

Responsive Care Takeaways for Using the Sense Pathways:

- The sense pathways can be used to affect emotions.

    Attitude: A willingness to learn the skills and use them.

    Attitude: Patience and the understanding that the activity of doing something together may be as valuable as any other reason, such as pain relief or relaxation.

- Essential oils trigger different emotions, depending on the oil involved.

    Action: Learn the various oils, actions and administration.

    Action: Use oils as carefully as you do drugs.

- Aromatherapy, via the use of essential oils in a diffuser, with or without water requires no effort on the part of the Person.

    Action: Set up a diffuser near, but out of reach of the Person. Use cool-mist when humidity will be helpful.

- Voluntary non-custodial touching is helpful in increasing self-worth and other positive emotions.
- Massage therapy uses both touch and smell to soothe the muscles and relax the brain. Acupuncture and acupressure relieve pain, negative feelings and stress. Acupuncture may be more effective but requires a trained professional.

  Action: Use lots of gentle but firm non-custodial touching. Add massage and acupressure therapy to soothe and provide quality together time. Consider acupuncture as needed.

- Aromatherapy can be combined with touch therapy.

  Action: Use essential oils with massage for more effectiveness.

- Sound therapy can improve cognition, speech and mobility for hours after a session.

  Action: Search out opportunities like Big and Loud© where the Person can experience musical and rhythmic activities.

- Visual stimulation uses light, color, shape and motion to stimulate and relax. Passive activities like looking at videos or photo albums can be entertaining.

  Action: Provide visual art opportunities for the Person. Choose passive activities that will stimulate only positive emotions.

28. Enhancing Activities

Enhancing activities are those that make a Person feel better about themself and their surroundings, while adding happiness and quality to one's life. We've known for years that a physically healthy lifestyle decreases the risk of dementia. It also decreases behaviors in people already living with dementia. Researchers now say that activities that foster *emotional* well-being are equally helpful. It makes sense. A Person tends to feel either "good" or "bad." Therefore, when a Person experiences positive feelings, such as happiness, contentment or fulfillment, the negative behavior-causing emotions are likely absent.

Mental Stimulation

Exercise instructors say about muscle tone: "Use it or lose it." Consider the brain a muscle. The more you use it, the better it works. Mentally active people tend to develop dementia later in life than do those who exercise their brain less. In people who have mild cognitive impairment already, mental activity appears to extend awareness, acting in this way "as well as any drug."[55]

Researchers think that mentally active people build up a "cognitive reserve" that masks encroaching dementia. When that reserve is gone, the course of the disorder accelerates, shortening the time of helplessness at end of life. This doesn't mean that a Person lives longer. More likely, the Person will have a better quality of life for a longer time followed by a short period of severe helplessness just prior to death.

Mental exercises may also improve one's ability to interact with others, help a Person maintain a sense of purpose and make life more interesting.

Mental stimulation does have limitations. It doesn't appear to have an effect on one's mood. Thus, it may not improve mood-related behaviors such as depression. However, it should still help those related to cognition, such as delusions and possibly, hallucinations.

Mental stimulation needs to be at least slightly challenging to be effective. However, as the Person's brain changes, what used to be easy becomes an acceptable challenge and what used to be challenging becomes unacceptably frustrating. Being responsive to the level of a Person's abilities will allow you to choose and adapt activities so that they provide challenges without frustration.

For better mental stimulation, try any or all of the following.

Take lessons. Has the Person always wanted to play tennis, play the piano or learn Spanish? Encourage giving it a try but don't make it stressful. The goal is to enjoy the challenge, not be perfect. Consider doing this as a couple. Do this early on, before the dementia makes doing new things no longer enjoyable.

Read a book. Read whatever is enjoyable. Although reading is often one of the first skills to go, stretch it out by using large print books or use an e-book and enlarge the print. As concentration skills decrease, the larger size print makes reading easier. A short attention span, and possibly a disappearing memory, can make lengthy books difficult even with large print. Choose books or magazine articles short enough to read at one sitting. Children's books have short stories in nice large print. Although the content is seldom right for adults, reading them to grandchildren might be a very enjoyable exercise. Find a list of books for adults here.[56]

Listen to someone else read. When reading is no longer possible—or even before, listen to someone read and then discuss what's been read. This exercises the brain twice—once when listening and again with the discussion. There's also a pleasant social aspect in reading aloud. During discussions, avoid questions. They require too much effort to answer and may change positive feelings to anxiety.

Larry was always a reader; he'd read four books to my one. He struggles with reading now...and I don't read out loud very well myself. I got him some audio books and he does like those. The problem with them is that I have to work the equipment for him. But then Amazon came out with their Echo. Now he just tells Echo to read to him and she does! -- Doris

Digital technology like this hands-free, voice controlled device adds a feeling of independence to a person's life.

Play solitary games: Do crossword puzzles, Sudoku, play solitaire or any of the many activities that take only one person. One skill may leave before another. For example, the Person may be able to do Sudoku with numbers long after he's stopped being able to do crossword or other word puzzles, or vice versa.

I'm so amazed. Larry can't even figure out how to work the smart phone to make a call but he can play solitaire on it. He knows how to find the game, how to play it and even when to start over. I don't know how he figured it out...I didn't tell him, but he does it. -- Doris

What a person can or can't do sometimes doesn't make sense. Larry has used a computer for years and knew how to play solitaire. He somehow was able to use those skills to master playing the game on a different device.

Play games with another person. This provides a chance for togetherness and socialization and allows the Person to be able to play the games longer. Even games meant for one person, like a crossword puzzle, can be done with two people.

Dean used to be able to play gin rummy and chess and beat me. When those games became too difficult, we enjoyed crossword puzzles together, and Chinese Checkers with pegs. When he could no longer focus on the pegs or small print, we played thinking games like Trivial Pursuit. We tried to answer questions as a team.[57] – Judy Towne Jennings in her book, Living with Lewy Body Dementia.

Although LBD eventually decreases cognitive skills even with the best of care, Dean and Judy didn't give up. They continued to find games both could enjoy. Start with a favorite. When it is no longer fun, either change the rules to make the game easier or find a different game.

Socialization

For years, experts have told us that exercise is better dementia treatment than drugs. Now they say that "socialization is every bit as good as exercise" for maintaining cognitive function. With LBD, this is directly connected to those unwanted behaviors which are often thinking related! In addition, socialization increases one's feeling of well-being, a strong positive feeling that also decreases behaviors. Use these suggestions to make an event successful:

- Ask family and friends to visit often, but only a few at a time. A Person can become overwhelmed when faced with more than a few people at a time.

- Encourage the Person to continue to participate in once beloved sports, games and hobbies. Adapt rules to simplify as needed, adding more socialization and less challenge.

- Add enjoyable events like going for ice cream (to the same place each time), to get the Person out with other people.
- Encourage the Person to continue to participate in social organizations that they have belonged to in the past. When there is a choice, choose smaller groups to attend.

Spirituality

Trust in a higher power decreases care partner stress and depression. The need for and value of a spiritual connection doesn't diminish with dementia. The practice of spirituality generates gratefulness, joy and awe while limiting worry and anxiety.

- Include spiritual routines such as saying grace at meals, meditation, prayer and a daily devotional reading in your daily life.

We've always said grace before meals and we still do. It's important to us but I'd do it even if it wasn't, just to maintain this ritual that Mom has had for so long. Mom has always read the Bible in the evening. Now part of her bedtime ritual is for me to read something from the Bible to her. She may tell me what to read. If not, I choose something that seems to fit our day. -- Shirley

- Encourage the Person to continue to attend the church or spiritual center of their choice. However, consider smaller gatherings, such as a study group rather than the larger church service.

Pets

There is such a thing as pet therapy, where the animals are trained to be well-mannered in uncomfortable settings.[58] However, such training is not necessarily needed in the home. A gentle well-behaved family pet can provide many benefits for a Person.

- The companionship and unconditional acceptance of a well-behaved, mild-mannered pet can decrease isolation, stress and depression.

- The care of a pet adds exercise, fun and meaningful activity while increasing the Person's feelings of self-worth.

- Pets aren't for everyone. Not only must the Person want to bond with the pet, but the care partner must accept that as dementia advances, the pet's care will be their responsibility.

- Some care facilities have resident pets or allow residents to have pets. Others invite service pets and their owners to visit.

Music and Rhythm

Music and rhythm work well as therapy, sometimes even better than physical or speech therapy for improving the ability to think, talk and move as discussed in the previous chapter, Using the Sense Pathways.

But music and rhythm can do much more. The documentary, *Alive Inside*,[59] tells of how social worker Dan Cohen, founder of Music and Memory, brought music into nursing homes and changed people's lives. Music can enhance our lives, feed our imagination and charge our emotions.

- When music or rhythm helps a Person to communicate or move better, their sense of well-being, feelings of adequacy and self-esteem all improve.

- Because of its close connection to both emotions and memory, music can be used for calming or energizing, for triggering memories of past emotions or for soothing painful thoughts.

- Music likes vary with the person and requires an individual playlist to be most effective.

- The effects of music and rhythm last long after the music stops. A Person who listens to music for an hour in the morning tends to be more alert and less restless for hours afterwards.

Being Creative

People who participate in cognitively stimulating activities and are socially engaged, have a better quality of life, and suffer less depression.[60] The positive effects of such an activity tend to last for hours after the event is over, leading to a happier, more content, less stressed Person--with fewer behaviors. There are multitudes of ways to encourage creativity, depending on the Person's personal preferences. Here are a couple of suggestions.

Improvisational theater, or improv, plays out in the here and now, with no memorized lines, no set story line, and no experience required.

Improv is a great tool for the care partner when dealing with a Person's irrational statements (see Chapter 12). However, improv acting can also be a creative and social way to stimulate the Person's mind. Guidelines for the participants are very similar to the ones for care partners who use improv techniques in their interactions with the Person:

- Say yes. Accept everything at face value. This is something that a Person does almost naturally!
- Encourage. Add something that moves the action on. The person with only mild cognitive impairment can usually do this well. A Person may need some coaching.
- Go with the flow. This will happen easily as the actors let go and play with the dialogue.
- Enjoy! Be careful to encourage fun and avoid criticism. Whatever they say is fine. That's the way improv is.

Most communities have improv groups and some groups offer special sessions for Persons. Ask at senior centers and your nearest Area Agency on Aging office.

Plant a garden. If getting down on the ground is difficult, use a raised garden plot. The Person can have fun playing in the dirt, seeing a flower grow and bloom, smelling the fresh air and experiencing the feel of working with the soil.

Carol was always a gardener. She can't get down on the ground anymore and so I built her a raised garden. She loves it when Carrie, our five-year-old granddaughter comes over and "helps" her. I don't know who gets dirtier, but I do know that she usually feels good for the rest of the day after a session in her little garden with Carrie. -- Harold

This is a good activity to do together or with others as Carol did with Carrie. (One child at a time, please!) Working on a mutual project adds a special feeling of communication without saying a word.

Do anything creative. If the Person has a craft or creative skill like painting or music, encourage them to continue doing it. Even though skills may degenerate as dementia advances, the enjoyment from being creative does not. Focus more on enjoyment than on performance. Several people with early dementia have written books. Others have used their art to communicate feelings even after speaking became difficult.

***

Responsive Care Takeaways for Enhancing Activities:

- A cognitively active person's built-up reserve provides a longer functional period with a shorter period of helplessness.

- Challenging but non-frustrating mental exercises improve interaction with others and add feelings of accomplishment.

    Attitude: A can-do attitude and a willingness to adapt helps the Person continue cognitively challenging activities.

    Actions:

    o Early on, encourage new experiences.

    o Make reading a part of the Person's routine, adapting easier books and then listening to you read as necessary.

    o Play games, adapting rules as necessary.

    o Socialization exercises the brain in a variety of ways, increasing well-being and decreasing behaviors. However, it can also be overwhelming.

    Action: Choose social opportunities that limit stimulation and demands on performance.

- Spiritual connections continue to be helpful for both Person and care partner.

    Action: Include familiar spiritual routines and pay attention to your own practices as well.

- Pets can provide companionship, unconditional acceptance and a sense of being useful, but do come with additional responsibilities for the care partner.

  Attitude: A sense of responsibility is necessary for pet ownership.

  Action: Choose to have a pet only if a) the Person enjoys animals and b) the care partner is willing to eventually be responsible for its care.

- Music and rhythm are closely connected to emotions and can calm or energize.

  Action: Make a playlist of the Person's favorite music and play it regularly.

- Being creative makes a Person feel happier, more worthwhile and content while relieving stress.

  Attitude: View fun rather than perfection as the creative goal.

  Action: Encourage improv acting, gardening, crafting, music or any other creative activity the Person might enjoy.

  Self-care: Make time and space for your own creative needs as well.

29. Sports, Games, Hobbies, Special Interests

Like the above creative activities, sports, games, hobbies and special interests that a Person has enjoyed for years can often be adapted so that they can continue to enjoy them well into their journey. The enjoyment and the feeling of accomplishment both serve to decrease stress and behaviors.

These activities also challenge more than one brain function, which increases their value as behavior-decreasing skills. Many include physical exercise. When any of the activities are done with another person or group, they include socialization. Most activities involve thinking of some kind, whether it is how far to hit the ball or which card to play, which exercises one's mental abilities.

Sports activities such as golf, tennis, bowling, and dancing are very helpful. Dancing also includes the use of music and rhythm and thus, is especially helpful.

We met at a dance. It has been one of our favorite activities for all of our marriage. We don't go out to dances anymore. The crowds on the floor and the low lights are uncomfortable for Gerry. But we still put on a favorite song and dance in the living room at home. It's amazing how mobile he can be when the music plays! And I notice that he often appears more alert for quite a while after we've quit dancing. -- Olivia

Music related activities, such as dancing, singing or playing an instrument can temporarily improve movement and clarity.

We square danced for several years after Annie was experiencing MCI. Eventually she couldn't keep up with the calls. – James

Annie's square dancing triggered the music pathway to her brain and temporarily improved clarity. Like any sport, it exercised several abilities at once, and in a fun way. Because square dancing requires the use of sequential learning, Annie eventually became unable to do it. However, she could likely have still done simple ballroom dancing where rhythm is more important than sequences. Rhythm lasts!

Table games, like playing cards or doing puzzles usually aren't very physical but they still generate the positive feelings that serve to decrease behaviors and exercise social and mental functions.

Steve and I play three hands of cards every morning right after breakfast. It's become a part of his routine. It's a time for us to do something together and we both value it. We've made the game simpler as his abilities changed but it still gives him a bit of a challenge and makes him feel better about himself. -- Rhonda

Hobbies, like stamp or antique collecting or scrapbooking are often creative as well. Like table games, they may not be physical, but they can still be challenging in other ways while being enjoyable.

Larry still gets a kick out of looking at the stamps he's been collecting since he was a kid. He hasn't added any stamps to his collection for a long time but he still loves to tell me stories about how he got this one or that one. -- Doris

Special interests, such as promoting a favorite charity, increase positive feelings of self-worth and add enjoyment.

Mom volunteered at the local animal shelter for years. She still does. She can't do much of the work anymore, but they can always use someone to cuddle the animals and give them some love. -- Shirley

Since the Person will mirror their companion's emotions, choose people who participate for fun, not for perfection. On the other hand, the companion should be willing to work at the Person's optimum ability so that there is challenge without undue stress.

Dementia eventually lowers abilities. That is no reason to quit an enjoyable activity. Instead, adapt, change the rules, do whatever you can to make it possible for the Person to continue. They might still play golf, but not keep score. Or play cards with relaxed rules. Or donate to a charity instead of attending a crowded charity function.

As the dementia progresses, the goals change. Put an emphasis on having fun, which is great therapy. Recognize that the challenge has changed from perfection to persistence.

I used to be a risk-taker, an "adrenalin junkie," seeking out thrills to fulfill my need for excitement. Now my disorder provides all the challenges I need. — Charles Schneider[61]

Watch the stress levels. Anytime these activities cause more stress than benefits, the advantages gained from the activity are lost. It may be time to adapt the rules—or change the focus.

***

Responsive Care Takeaways for Sports, Games, Hobbies, and Special Interests:

- Sports, games, hobbies and special interests often include more than one way to challenge brain function, combining exercise, socialization and mental stimulation.
- Activities should challenge without being overwhelming.
- Participating in these activities adds quality of life.

   Attitude: A positive attitude and a willingness to adapt as needed facilitate the Person's enjoyment of these activities.

   Action: Encourage the Person to continue enjoyable activities, adapting the rules as needed and changing the goal from perfection to persistence and sometimes, from action to reminiscing.

Summing It Up

Being a Person living with dementia is not easy. It's not something anyone chooses. Bodies become less manageable, normal routes of communication become more difficult, thinking becomes more concrete and confusion more common. They cannot change but the care partner can. Responsive care is all about recognizing this and finding ways to respond with changes that make the lives of both Person and care partner much more pleasant.

Yes, it is all up to the care partner, who feels overwhelmed already. However, with knowledge of how the dementia-damaged brain works, you can choose attitudes and actions that support the Person's need to feel accepted, heard, safe, useful and content. When you take the time and effort to respond instead of react, you will find the quality of both of your lives improved.

Responsive care also includes knowing that while drugs may be the easiest way to deal with behaviors, they can often cause more problems than they solve. In response to this, a care partner must find alternative options that best meet the needs of their particular Person. This often time-consuming effort will pay for itself with more peace of mind, a happier Person and more chances for togetherness.

***

- Truly believe that a healthy, rested, happy care partner is your best caregiving tool and allow time to make that so for you.

- Educate yourself about dementia, how it damages the brain and what's left to work with.

- Know about drug sensitivity and how to avoid it.

- Search out and use alternative behavior management methods.

- Learn to avoid, decrease or remove the Person's stress triggers.

- Recognize behaviors as stress-related efforts to communicate.

- Accept the Person's reality and let go of your expectations.

- Take your time and relax.

- Use the Person's ability to mirror to guide them into happy changes.

- Use improv acting to make joining a Person's reality easier.

- Know how negative and positive emotions drive behavior and use it often.

- Copiously use apologies to defuse negativity and compliments to foster positivity but always with sincerity.

- Try reorienting a Person with hallucinations or mis-identifications by using a different sense pathway.

- Exercise and socialization promote good mental health prior to dementia and decrease dementia symptoms. Good nutrition and mental stimulation also help.

- Activities that use multiple ways of stimulating mental health are more effective than those that stimulate only one.

- Continue spiritual practices and other activities important to the Person for as long as possible, adapting as necessary.

- Keep a record of what works and what doesn't.

- Don't forget to add humor and having fun to both of your routines.

Resources

General Caregiver Information

Assist Guide Information Center. (agis.com) Excellent site with checklists, databases, information, and other caregiver support.

Caregiver Action Network. (caregiveraction.org). Their Caregiver Toolkit contains many guides such as Managing Medication or Financial Planning. 202-772-5050.

Disability.gov.(dol.gov/odep/topics/disability.htm) Federal website of comprehensive disability-related government resources.

*Family Caregiver Alliance. (*caregiver.org*)* One of the best caregiver sources on the internet. Find databases for a multitude of local resources by state in the right hand panel (with map). 800-445-8106.

National Association of Area Agencies on Aging. (n4a.org) Offers a variety of services to seniors. Most areas will have local offices. 202-872-8888.

SeniorLiving.org A comprehensive directory of senior living options and more. Includes a section on research with interesting facts about seniors and helpful guides for variety of subjects including government aid (see next item).

A Guide to Government aid for Seniors.
(seniorliving.org/research/government-aid/) Offers a
thorough review of US government services available to
seniors. Sponsored by Seniorliving.org. Be sure to scroll to
the end for additional resources.

Dementia Care Programs that advocate fewer drugs

Teepa Snow: Positive Approach to Brain Change.
(teepasnow.com) A great source of ideas for dementia care,
stress management and general caregiving. Offers a variety
of valuable training for care partners and staff. Since we
have monitored a training class, we can personally
recommend Teepa Snow's work.

> *YouTube videos.* *(youtube.com/user/teepasnow/videos)*
> Free Teepa Snow videos on a wide variety of dementia
> related subjects.

DICE Approach.
(programforpositiveaging.org/diceapproach/) **D**escribe,
Investigate, **C**reate, **E**valuate. Free interactive trainings
provide caregivers "a better understanding of the causes of
BPSD and teach how to apply the DICE Approach when
the behaviors occur." University of Michigan Program for
Positive Aging.

Eden Alternative. (edenalt.org) Dementia Care Beyond
Drugs. Through education, consultation, and outreach, this
group offers "person-directed principles and practices that
support the unique needs of different living environments."
Based on the book *Dementia Beyond Drugs, Changing the
Culture of Care,* by G. Allen Power, MD, available on
Amazon.

Improv/Dementia Groups

In the Moment. *(in-themoment.net/training-programs.html)* A well recognized program aimed at improving "the quality of life for all dementia warriors." Offers videos, podcasts and articles about using improv with dementia.

TEDMED videos.

(tedmed.com/speakers/show?id=526373) Seven speeches about different ways to use improv techniques with people living with dementia. By *In the Moment* founders, Karen Strobbe and Mondy Carter.

Dementia RAW. *(dementiaraw.com/programs)* A training program offered by Silver Dawn Training Institute. Uses a combination of improv techniques and empathy to "simplify communication." In the past, has offered a Dementia Communication Essentials Program for Family Caregivers, $25 online, $50 in person. Check the website for future offerings. Also offers a book, Start with YES!, by Cathy Braxton and Tami Neumann. Sold on their website and on Amazon.

The Memory Ensemble. *(brain.northwestern.edu/support/QoL%20Programs/memory_ensemble.html)* An eight-week long theater intervention program for people with early stage dementia, using improv acting "to provide challenging and supportive creative learning opportunities to improve quality of life." A collaboration between Northwestern Michigan University and the Lookingglass Theater Company. Check the website for dates and articles.

Alternative Therapy Information

LBDtools.com. Our own website, which has a large section on a variety of alternative options for use with people living with dementia, written by our alternative therapy consultant, Regina Hucks.

Complementary and Alternative Treatments for Dementia, by Esther Heerema, MSW, on the Very Well Health website, *(verywellhealth.com/complementary-and-alternative-therapies-for-dementia-98671)* advertizes that it makes an effort to offer unbiased information. Heerma's article provides a good overview of non-drug options that can be used with or without drugs for people living with dementia.

Whole New Mom. *(wholenewmom.com)* "Research-based healthy living you can trust." Adrienne wrote a well thought out six-part blog on essential oils, how to choose them, which company she prefers and why. To access, click on the search icon in the menu bar and write "essential oil."

An Introductory Guide to 1000's of Uses for Essential Oils. *(sustainablebabysteps.com/uses-for-essential-oils.html)* Sustainable Baby Steps website. Lists oils alphabetically with their functions. A good basic reference. Identifies the qualities of a "good oil" but doesn't name a brand.

Acupressure for Beginners. *(exploreim.ucla.edu/self-care /acupressure-and-common-acupressure-points/)* An Explore Integrative Medicine blog from the UCLA Center for East-West Medicine. Explains how acupressure works and offers some basic directions for use. Is not specific to dementia.

The Role of Massage Therapy in Dementia Care, A *Women in Bodywork* blog by Ann Catlin. *(massagetoday.com/mpacms/mt/article.php?id=15057)* The blog provides a good overview of how you can use massage to help a person living with dementia feel among other things, less pain and anxiety.

Drug Information

Drugs.com. A drug interaction checker lists all interactions for a single drug with severity as well as checking for interactions between an individualized list of drugs. By signing in, you can accumulate information from successive searches. Also offers a pill checker with photos of pills.

LBDA Medical Alert Wallet Card. *(lbda.org/content/lbd-medical-alert-wallet-card)* Carry this card with you everywhere.

Publications for Professionals. *(lbda.org/physicians)* A list of articles and checklists designed especially for professionals. Good articles to copy and give to doctors and other medical staff

Treating Psychosis in LBD. *(lbda.org/go/ER)* Download this and add it to your Emergency Room packet.

Anticholinergic drug lists. To access the following two sites, enter the *complete title* into a search engine.

The Revised Beers Criteria (Medication List). Revised by the American Geriatric Society in 2012, this extensive list shows drugs by use, and quality of evidence but not brand names.

Anticholinergics and the Elderly-Detail document.
Compiled in 2011 from several other sources, this scale
shows brand names, drugs uses and levels of
anticholinergic risk.

Medical Assistance Programs

Medicare.gov. The Official U.S. Government Site for People
with Medicare.

Benefits.gov. This official government benefits website is a
free, confidential tool that helps individuals find
government benefits they may be eligible to receive.

Social Security Administration. *(ssa.gov)* The toll-free
number is live 7AM to 7PM EST, Monday to Friday.
Recorded information and services are available 24 hours a
day. The website provides a wealth of information and
resources including many databases and publications. 800-
772-1213.

Veterans Administration. *(va.gov)* Site provides information
on VA benefits and services such as Aid & Attendance.
800-827-1000.

Hilarity for Charity. *(hilarityforcharity.org)* An organization
that raises money for grants for dementia caregiver
assistance. Use the online email contact form to apply for
a grant for help with home care.

Disease Specific Support Organization

Lewy Body Dementia

Lewy Body Dementia Association *(lbda.org)* An excellent
source of LBD Caregiver forums, information and support.
Many local support groups. Caregiver line: 844-311-0587.
Office: 404-975-2322.

Caring Spouses Group *(groups.io/g/LBDCaringSpouses)* A private group limited to spouses of LBD patients. To join the group, use this email link: LBDCaringSpouses+subscribe@groups.io

Lewy Body Dementia Support Group, Facebook. *(facebook.com)* Enter "Lewy Body Dementia Support" in the Facebook search box. A closed group, easy to join. For anyone interested in LBD.

Alzheimer's Disease

Alzheimer's Association. *(alz.org)* Nationwide Local Chapters and Caregiver Support Groups. Helpline: 800-272-3900.

Alzheimer's Foundation of America. *(alzfdn.org)* Social Worker Helpline: 866-232-8484. (Also available via Skype, live chat or email.)

***Alzheimer's Disease Education and Referral (ADEAR) Center*.** *-(nia.nih.gov/alzheimers)* Sponsored by the National Institute of Health, this site provides a current, comprehensive, unbiased source of information about Alzheimer's disease.

Frontotemporal Disorders

The Association for Frontotemporal Degeneration. *(theaftd.org)* Provides accurate information, compassion and hope when lives are touched by any type of FTD. Helpline email: info@theaftd.org. Helpline: 866-507-7222

Early-Onset Dementia

Early LBD Virtual Support Group. *(lbda.org/forum)* A private sub-forum on the LBDA.org website for those with early LBD. In the Living with LBD section.

Early-Onset Caregiver's Support Group. *(groups.yahoo.com)* Enter "Early Onset Caregiver" in the Search Groups box at the top of the page to access group. A private online support group for caregivers of people with early onset dementia of any kind.

Memory People, Facebook group. *(facebook.com)* Enter "Memory People" in the search box. Started by Early Onset AD patient Rick Phelps. A private place where patients with early dementia and their caregivers share experiences and concerns.

Glossary

Note: Words that are italicized are defined in this glossary.

abstract thinking: thinking that uses executive skills to reason and develop concepts, including time-related ideas, levels of relationship and comparisons.

accept: To agree to a situation without attempting to change or protest it. Acceptance and belief are not the same--one can accept without believing. Acceptance is aimed at utility and function rather than truth.

acetylcholine: A *neurotransmitter* involved with memory, sleep, muscle movement, and automatic functions such as heart rate and body secretions. Often targeted by *Lewy bodies*.

active dreams: Care partner's name for *REM sleep behavior disorder*. When a chemical switch in the brain that turns off mobility during dreams is damaged, a person thrashes their limbs about, talks and can even be unintentionally violent while asleep.

activities of daily living (ADL): Basic daily activities necessary for independent living. Includes eating, bathing, dressing, toileting, transferring and maintaining *continence*.

acupressure: Using finger pressure on the bodily sites used in acupuncture to mildly stimulate nerve impulses to relieve pain and promote healing. Not as effective as acupuncture but does not require a professional.

acupuncture: The insertion of the tips of needles by a trained professional into the skin at specific points to stimulate nerve impulses to relieve pain and promote healing.

adult day care: A program that provides a few hours of supervised care with activities such as meals, socializing and songfests one or more times a week, while providing respite time for a care partner.

adverse drug reaction: Unexpected, unwanted or dangerous reaction to a drug, usually just the opposite of the usual effect. The onset of the adverse reaction may be sudden or develop over time. Also termed adverse effect or adverse event.

agitation: Excessive motor activity associated with a feeling of inner *tension.* Can be seen as verbal and physical aggression, active resistance to care, pacing, fidgeting, hand wringing, pulling of clothes and the inability to sit still.

alpha-synuclein: A normal protein present in the central nervous system. When damaged (misfolded), clumps of alpha-synuclein protein can become *Lewy bodies.*

alternative options: Non-drug remedies, interventions and *therapies.* Can be used alone or in combination with drug *therapy.*

alternative therapy: Therapy other than traditional, drug-related *therapies.* Usually refers to *sense*-related techniques like *aromatherapy* and *massage.*

alternative/optional therapy: Other-than-drug treatment of disease or disorders, by some remedial, rehabilitating, or curative process. May be used alone or in combination with drugs.

Alzheimer's disease: The most common progressively degenerative *dementia*. Because thinking ability may not be impaired until late in the disease, *dementia related behaviors* may also be later.

ambulatory: Able to walk about; not bed-ridden and do not need a wheelchair to get around.

anesthetic: Drug action that reduces pain.

anti-anxiety drugs: (tranquilizers) Drugs used to treat *anxiety, agitation*, nervousness and *tension* and as *muscle relaxants*. Most are also *anticholinergics*.

anticholinergic: Drug action that reduces the effect of *acetylcholine*, the same *neurotransmitter* that *Lewy bodies* attack. Includes *muscle relaxants, anti-anxiety drugs, sedatives, antipsychotic drugs* and drugs that treat *Parkinson's* symptoms.

anti-convulsants: Drugs used to control convulsions.

antidepressants: Drugs used to treat depression. (Celexa, Desyrel, Paxil, Prozac, selective serotonin reuptake inhibitors, Zoloft)

antipsychotic drugs: (*neuroleptic* drugs) Drugs approved for treating *psychotic* symptoms in *diseases* such as schizophrenia and may be used off label with *dementia* symptoms such as *hallucinations, delusions* and *agitation*. Most are *anticholinergics*.

anxiety: Feelings of *unease, tension, worry* and *apprehension*. Often accompanied by compulsive behavior.

apathy: A lack of *motivation* and the inability to *initiate* activities or conversations.

271

apprehension: Feelings of anxiety, *unease*, nervousness or worry, the fear that something bad or unpleasant will happen.

aromatherapy: The use of essential oils to improve physical and mental well-being.

atrophy: Decrease in size or wasting away of a body part of tissue.

attention deficit: Difficulty in sustaining attention resulting in impulsive behavior and excessive activity.

autonomic functions: Involuntary functions regulated by the *autonomic nervous system*. Includes the activities of the heart, the gastrointestinal tract, the urinary tract, and the glands.

autonomic nervous system: Part of the nervous system which regulates key functions of the body. *Lewy bodies* can affect this system and cause a slowing down of *autonomic functions.*

behaviors: A person's actions. Used in this book as shorthand for "*dementia-related behaviors.*"

benzodiazepine: Drugs used as *anti-anxiety drugs, muscle relaxants*, and anti-convulsants. Are usually *anticholinergic.*

Big and Loud© (also called Lee Silverman Voice Training): Evidence-based speech, physical and occupational therapies for people with Parkinson's and other conditions. LSVT Big and Loud© offers groups to help participants learn to use existing abilities better, to speak more clearly, to move better and even to think better. Website: https://www.lsvtglobal.com/

black box warning: FDA required warning on all antipsychotic product packaging indicating that the use of antipsychotics in the elderly is linked to increased risk of serious illness and death.

burnout: physical, *emotion*al and mental exhaustion so great that it is difficult to be positive and caring.

Capgras syndrome: The *delusional* belief that a person or pet is really an impostor or clone of the "real" person or pet.

care partner: A *care* person/*care*giver who recognizes that *dementia care* works best as partnership between them and the *Person*.

care person: Preferred term for anyone caring for a *Person* living with *dementia*.

care: The physical responsibility for a Person living with dementia. Includes *home health, residential, palliative, hospice* and *long term*.

caregiver support group: A place where *care partners* can share experiences and concerns, build friendships and feel refreshed.

caregiver: General term for anyone caring for a *Person* living with *dementia* or other illness. Limited use in this book due to its connotation that *care* is given, rather than it being a *team* effort.

chronic: Pertaining to a long-lasting symptom, usually related to a long-lasting disease.

clinical trials: Trials to evaluate the effectiveness and safety of medications or medical devices by monitoring their effects on large groups of people.

cognition: The process of being able to use one's *abstract thinking* abilities to be aware and to know, think, learn and judge.

cognitive abilities: Skills used to facilitate memory, executive *functions, perception*, control *impulses* and *communicate.*

cognitive fluctuations: Fluctuations of the severity of *dementia* symptoms, with some periods of time of appearing nearly normal fluctuating with periods of much more severe symptoms. Common with Lewy body *dementia.*

communication: An interaction where words, actions and feelings are based on the same reality.

compassion fatigue: Extreme state of *stress* resulting in feelings of hopelessness, indifference, pessimism and lack of *empathy.*

compassionate: Having sympathy and concern for the Person's pain, needs and wishes.

concrete thinking: Primitive thinking based on material information derived from the *dementia-related behaviors* in the here and now.

conscious choice: A decision made by taking the time to use *abstract thinking* to evaluate a situation and decide upon a response.

continence: The ability to control functions of elimination. Lack results in *urinary or fecal incontinence.*

deficit: Physical and/or *cognitive* skill or ability that a *Person* once had but has lost, has difficulty with, or can no longer perform.

delayed gratification: The ability to resist an immediate reward and wait for a later, often larger or better treat.

delusion of misidentification: *A delusional* belief that a person or place has been replaced by an impostor.

Capgras syndrome and *location delusions* are both *delusion*s of misidentification.

delusion: The false or irrational belief, usually based on the first information the brain receives about an event or person. Includes *Capgras Syndrome, paranoia,* and results in *delusional accusations, locations* and *stories*.

delusional accusation: An accusation, based on a *delusion*al belief usually of theft, infidelity or abandonment.

delusional location: (*reduplicative par-amnesia*) The *delusional* belief that a place or object has been replaced by a substitute.

delusional story: An often grandiose story of something the Person *delusionally* believes they have experienced or seen.

dementia care: *Care* provided for Person living with dementia. Includes *home health, hospice, long term, palliative, residential* and *respite.*

dementia drug: Drug used to treat the cognitive aspects of dementia. Two basic types, each acting on a different *neurotransmitter*. Three, Aricpet, Exelon and Razadyne, act on *acetylcholine*. Namenda acts on glutamate.

dementia: A decline in cognition (mental ability) severe enough to interfere with two or more activities of daily living.

dementia-related behaviors: (or just "behaviors") The Person living with dementia's often disruptive responses to *perceptual*, thought and *mood* disturbances.

dementia-sensitive drug: Drug that may cause *drug sensitivity* when taken by a *Person* living with *dementia*. Includes most *antipsychotics, anti-anxiety drugs, sedatives* and *anticholinergics.*

depressant: (*sedative hypnotic*) A drug or substance that depresses brain activity, resulting in calmness, slowed breathing, reduction in anxiety, muscle relaxation, and sleepiness. Usually *anticholinergic.* Includes *benzodiazepines*, alcohol, *anesthetics*, and *anticonvulsants*.

depression: a persistent feeling of sadness and loss of interest in activities once enjoyed. Can be *chronic*, as when caused by a disease such as dementia or *situational,* as when a person receives their diagnosis.

diffuser: a device that disperses essential oils into the surrounding air. Used with *aromatherapy*.

disease/disorder: A group of symptoms with a common cause and outcome. Disease is normally used when the cause and outcome are clear. Disorder is normally used when they are less clear, but both are often used clinically for the same conditions.

disinhibition: Acting upon an impulse, urge or temptation without considering consequences or social conventions.

dopamine: A *neurotransmitter* involved in pleasure, motivation, *cognition* and *mobility*. Often targeted by Lewy bodies, leading to apathy or Parkinson's loss of mobility.

drug sensitivity: The reaction to a normal dose as though it were an overdose—sometimes a huge overdose. Varies greatly with each Person and each drug.

dry mouth: Condition of not having enough saliva to keep the mouth wet, caused by inadequately functioning salivary glands.

elder law attorney: Attorney who practices in the area of elder law which focuses on issues typically affecting older adults.

elderly: (geriatric) Pertaining to people approximately age 65 and older. This population is usually more drug-sensitive.

emotion: (feelings) State of mind triggered by the *senses*, situations or people, usually triggered prior to *abstract thinking*. Can be *positive, negative* or *residual*.

empathetic responding: Responding to a *Person* in ways they can hear and accept.

empathy deficit: Inability to feel *empathy*, which can appear as indifference or self-centeredness.

empathy: The ability to see events and experiences from another person's viewpoint, imagine what that person is feeling but know that the feeling is theirs and not yours.

engage: To occupy, attract or involve one's interest

essential oils: Highly concentrated extracts from flowers, leaves, and other plant parts.

excessive daytime sleepiness: A *dementia*-related tendency to fall asleep intermittently during the day.

executive skills: Those used for judgment and reasoning, decision making and choices, organizing and sequencing, comparing and generalizing, connecting cause and effect.

fecal incontinence: Inability to control the expelling of feces.

flexibility: The ability to let go of the old and adapt, to cope with changes and think about tasks in creative ways.

geriatric: Pertaining to the *elderly*.

guilt: An *emotion* triggered by perceived personal wrongdoing that becomes destructive when used as a method for trying to control the past.

Haldol: Trade name for haloperidol: A traditional antipsychotic drug. Particularly dangerous for LBD patients.

hallucination: The *perception* of something in any of the five *senses* that is not really there. Often an early LBD symptom.

hand-eye coordination: Cognitive function related to the combination of visual and spatial awareness and ability.

home health: Service that provides in-home *care*.

hospice: Program that provides *care* to Persons near the end of life. Focus is on comfort rather than recovery. Covered by Medicare.

illusion: The *perception* of something real as something else, such as a small box as a small animal.

improv acting: Putting one's own *reality* on hold--leaving it off the stage--and playing your given part with conviction in the Person's drama.

improvisational (improv) theater: A form of live theater where the dialogue, story, and characters are created by the actors as the action unfolds in present time.

impulsivity: Acting without thought.

inflexibility: Rigid attitude with an inability to see a need to change, often caused by immobilizing *negative emotions* like fear and worry.

initiate: To begin or start an activity. An ability that fades with *dementia.*

insomnia: Difficulty getting to sleeping or staying asleep.

interaction: talking, looking, sharing, or engaging in any kind of action that involves two or more people. May or may not be based on the same reality.

irritability: An over-reaction to stimuli, as in the sensitiveness of skin irritability or a Person's emotional behaviors such as anger, impatience or anxiety.

LBD: Common anagram for *Lewy body dementia*, Lewy *body disease* or *Lewy body disorder*. Because LBD is more than dementia, we use the anagram LBD almost exclusively so that you can choose which of these YOU want to call it.

Lewy bodies: Microscopic round clumps of normal proteins that have become damaged, so that they clump together inside neurons, causing more damage. Present in REM Sleep Behavior Disorder, Parkinson's Disease and LBD.

Lewy body dementia: (Lewy body *disease* , Lewy body *disorder* or just *LBD*): The second most common progressively degenerative dementia. Affects *cognition*, *mobility* and *autonomic functions*.

Lewy-sensitive drug: One that may cause *drug sensitivity* when taken by a Person living with LBD. The effects vary greatly with each Person although some drugs are more likely to be Lewy-sensitive than others. Includes most *antipsychotics*, *anti-anxiety drugs*, *sedatives* and *anticholinergics*.

long term care: Program that provides ongoing skilled nursing. Not usually covered by Medicare.

loved one: A family member or *care partner*'s title for their *Person* living with *dementia*. This term is less appropriate for professional *care persons* but we recognize its gentle validity. Feel free to substitute it at will!

mandala: (sacred circle) A complex abstract design that is usually circular in form, with an identifiable center point.

martyrdom: The act of putting another's needs first, at the expense of one's own to the extent that it becomes damaging.

massage: Kneading or applying pressure to body tissues to improve circulation, soothe and relax.

melatonin: Natural herbal used to treat sleep disorders.

memory: The mental capacity of storing, encoding, retaining and retrieving information.

mindful listening: Listening with eyes, ears, touch and *empathy*. Being aware of the whole *Person* and looking past their behaviors to discover the original message.

mobility: The ability to move and the amount of movement.

moods: *Emotion*al states that can last a long time. Longer lasting negative moods such as *depression* are often considered to be disorders.

motivation: The ability to move forward.

muscle relaxants: Drugs used to decrease muscle spasms, cramps and pain. Many are *anticholinergic*.

Namenda: (memantine hydrochloride) A *dementia* drug often used with other *dementia drugs*. It acts on the *neurotransmitter* glutamate.

negative emotions: Feelings such as fear, anger and frustration act as motivators that trigger *dementia-related behaviors*.

nerve: A bundle of *neurons* that uses chemical and electrical signals to send and receive information from one body part to another.

neuro: Prefix meaning brain, as in *neurotransmitter*, *neuron*, neuropathy, neurologist or neurosurgeon.

neuroleptic malignant syndrome: Rare, possibly fatal, expression of *neuroleptic sensitivity*, with confusion, high fever, unstable blood pressure, muscular rigidity, and *stress* dysfunction.

neuroleptic sensitivity: (*drug sensitivity*) Negative reaction to an *antipsychotic drug* with symptoms such as rigidity,

immobility, loss of balance, difficulties with posture, sedation, and more.

neurologist: A physician specializing in *neurology*--diseases of the brain.

neuron: Nerve cell used for passing information.

neurotransmitter: A *neuro*-chemical that transfers information from one *neuron* (brain cell) to another.

nightmares: Dreams arousing feelings of intense fear, horror, or distress.

non-drug options: (*alternative options*) Therapies, techniques and interventions that do not use drugs but may be used in combination with drugs.

nonverbal cues: Gestures, facial expressions and even *dementia-related behaviors* used to express needs and wishes.

occupational therapy: *Therapy* that helps a Person adapt and compensate for lost daily living skills and to maintain feelings of usefulness and self-worth.

off-label drug: A drug that is prescribed for a different reason than that for which it has been approved by the Federal Drug Administration.

over-stimulation: (Sense overload) More stimuli than the brain can process.

palliative care: Program that provides *care* focusing on comfort rather than recovery to people who do not yet qualify for *hospice care*. Not covered by Medicare, but usually reasonably priced.

paranoia: A paranoid or *delusion*al fear, or paranoia, of something or someone.

Parkinson's disease: A Lewy body disorder, characterized by movement dysfunctions. Often a precursor to Lewy body *dementia*.

perception: A mental impression of what is sensed by any of the five *senses*.

Person (with a capital P): The Person living with *dementia*. A person (without a capital P) is anyone, a person who may or may not be living with *dementia*.

person-centered: Respectful of and responsive to an individual's preferences, needs, and values.

physical therapy: *Therapy* that helps the *Person* use remaining physical abilities and strengths to improve muscles, balance and mobility, manage pain and prevent falls to regain or improve their physical abilities.

positive emotions: *Emotions* such as happiness and comfort can calm and relax.

psychiatrist: Physician who specializes in the prevention, diagnosis, and treatment of mental illness. A *geriatric* psychiatrist specializes in the psychiatry of the elderly.

psychological therapy/counseling: The process or talking to a trained *therapist* or counselor about *emotional* and mental problems and relationships in order to understand and improve the way one feels, behaves and *interact*s.

psychosis: The presence of symptoms, such as *delusions* or *hallucinations*, that indicate an impaired contact with *reality*.

reacting: Making an immediate, usually negative, response to a situation, often without considering the consequences.

reality: What an individual believes is true. When a *Person* believes something is true, this is their *reality* and it can't be changed.

reduplicative par-amnesia: see *delusional location*.

REM sleep behavior disorder: Sleep disorder in which a dreamer physically acts out their dreams, sometimes unintentional violence to bed partner.

REM: Rapid eye movement, which shows that a person is dreaming.

residential care: Program that provides *care* in a residential facility. *Assisted living*, *memory care* and skilled nursing are all types of residential care.

residual emotions: *Emotions* left over in the brain from a previous experience.

respite care: Planned or emergency short-term care for the Persons living with dementia that provides respite for their care partners.

respite: A break from a difficult, exhausting or *emotion*ally draining situation.

responding/being responsive. Making a thought-out response to a situation vs. reacting.

responsive care: Informed, *person-centered*, *empathetic* and *accepting dementia* care, where the *care partner* also gives self-care a high priority.

rigidity: Increased muscle tone in neck, arms or legs. A typical symptom of *Parkinson's disease*.

sedative: Drug action that assists sleep by depressing the central nervous system. May cause serious side effects for Persons living with dementia. Often very addictive.

sedatives: Drugs used as sleeping aids or with anxiety. Many are *anticholinergic*.

selective attention: Focusing on particular areas of *sensory* experience, rather than passively absorbing everything.

self-care: A care partner's most important tool. Making sure one's ability to function is not damaged by neglect, overwork or *emotion*al distress.

senses/sensory: Sight, smell, hearing, taste, and touch; faculties by which the brain receives external stimuli.

showtime: Appearing better than normal in the presence of a person other than the care partner.

situational: Pertaining to a symptom caused by a situation. A situational symptom can improve when the situation or the *perception* of that situation improves.

sleep apnea: Temporary stoppage of breathing during sleep, often resulting in daytime sleepiness.

socialization: Interacting with other people. An activity that lowers risk of dementia and improved the lives of Persons living with dementia.

sound therapy: An alternative *therapy* using sound, music, rhythm and vibrations to improve *mood* and clarity.

stimulus/stimuli: Something that causes a body response. Most are delivered by one or more of the five senses.

stress management: Preventing, decreasing or removing *stressors*.

stress overload: Amount of *stress* greater than one's threshold.

stress threshold: Amount of *stress* tolerated without damage.

stress, chronic: Stress that lasts long past the immediate danger and is internalized as physical discomfort or damage.

stress: Physical, mental or *emotion*al pressure or *tension*.

stressors: Anything that causes *emotion*al, mental or physical discomfort or distress.

symptomatic treatment: Treatment which affects only symptoms, but not their cause.

team member: One of two or more people who are working together towards a common goal.

tension: Feelings of emotional strain, with an inability to relax.

therapeutic fibbing: Speaking from the *Person's reality* rather than your own in order to avoid increased anxiety and agitation.

therapist: A person with professional training in the art of their chosen field.

therapy: The treatment of disease or disorders, by some remedial, rehabilitating, or curative process. Includes drug, *occupational, physical, psychological therapies* and *alternative/optional therapies* such as *aroma, sound, speech* and *touch.*

touch therapy: Using one's hands to stimulate the tactile pathways to the brain. May or may not involve the use of *essential oils, massage, acupuncture, or acupressure.*

unease: Feelings of mental discomfort, worry, dissatisfaction or embarrassment.

urinary incontinence: Inability to control the start of urination.

worry: An *emotion* triggered by concern about a future event that becomes destructive when used to try to control the future.

References

[1] **Kim H** (2016) Behavioral and Psychological Symptoms of Dementia. Ann Psychiatry Ment Health 4(7):1086. https://www.jscimedcentral.com/Psychiatry/psychiatry-4-1086.pdf

[2] **Steinberg, M., & Lyketsos, C.** (2012). Atypical Antipsychotic Use In Patients With Dementia: Managing Safety Concerns. The American Journal of Psychiatry, 169(9), 900–906. doi.org/10.1176/appi.ajp.2012.12030342

[3] **Lewy Body Dementia Association.** (2015) Medications Glossary: Drug Classes and Medications. LBDA.org. http://www.lbda.org/sites/default/files/medication_glossary_2015.pdf

[4] **Brooks M.** (2018) New Practice Guidelines on Antipsychotic Use in Dementia. Medscape. May 03, 2016. https://www.medscape.com/viewarticle/862795

[5] **Fernandes J.** (2017) Study Reviews Use of Acadia's Nuplazid as Treatment for Psychosis Linked to Parkinson's Disease. Parkinson's News Today. https://parkinsonsnewstoday.com/2017/06/19/parkinsons-therapy-nuplazid-pimavanserin-reviewed-as-treatment-for-psychosis/

[6] **Ellison J.** (2016) Depression and Alzheimer's Disease. Bright Focus Foundation. https://www.brightfocus.org/alzheimers/article/depression-and-alzheimers-disease

[7] **Greene J.** (2005) Apraxia, agnosias, and higher visual function abnormalities. J Neurol Neurosurg Psychiatry 2005;76:v25-v34 doi:10.1136/jnnp.2005.081885. http://jnnp.bmj.com/content/76/suppl_5/v25.full

[8] **Alzheimer's Society.** (2012) Sight, perception and hallucinations in dementia. Alzheimer's Fact Sheets. https://www.alzheimers.org.uk/download/downloads/id/3369/sight_perception_and_hallucinations_in_dementia.pdf

[9] **Stone A.** (2014) Smell Turns Up in Unexpected Places. The New York Times. Oct. 13, 2014. https://www.nytimes.com/2014/10/14/science/smell-turns-up-in-unexpected-places.html?_r=1

[10] **D. Lynn.** An Old Flame, A poem in Whitworth H and Whitworth J., A Caregiver's Guide to Lewy Body Dementia. 2011. Demos Health Publishing.

[11] **Hudson T** (2017) May 7, 2017. Beware of "Showtime": Temporary Normalcy in Social Situations. In the full article: Have a New Lewy Body Dementia Diagnosis? http://www.lewybodydementia.ca/new-lewy-body-dementia-diagnosis/#Showtime

[12] **Goetz CG, et al.** (2006). The malignant course of "benign" hallucinations in Parkinson's Disease. Archives of Neurology 63:713-716. http://www.ncbi.nlm.nih.gov/pubmed/16682540

[13] **Alzheimer's Society blog.** (2017) Is there a link between stress and dementia risk? Saturday, April 15, 2017. https://blog.alzheimers.org.uk/research/stress-and-dementia/

[14] **Despues D.** (1999) Stress and Illness. California State University, Northridge. Spring, 1999. http://www.csun.edu/~vcpsy00h/students/illness.htm

[15] **Changing Minds.** (2002) Fight-or-Flight Reaction. Changing Minds.org. (2002-2015) http://changingminds.org/explanations/brain/fight_flight.htm

[16] **Collingwood J.** (2007) The Physical Effects of Long-Term Stress. PsychCentral. http://psychcentral.com/lib/the-physical-effects-of-long-term-stress/

[17] **Eres R, et al.** (2015). Anatomical differences in empathy related brain areas: A voxel-based morphometry study. Front. Hum. Neurosci. Conference Abstract: XII International Conference on Cognitive Neuroscience (ICON-XII). doi: 10.3389/conf.fnhum.2015.217.00187 http://www.frontiersin.org/10.3389/conf.fnhum.2015.217.00187/event_abstract

[18] **Heitz C, et al.** (2015) Cognitive and affective theory of mind in Lewy body dementia: A preliminary study. Rev Neurol (Paris). 2015 Apr;171(4):373-81. doi: 10.1016/j.neurol.2015.02.010. Epub 2015 Apr 3. http://www.ncbi.nlm.nih.gov/pubmed/25847396

[19] **Smith M, et. al.** (2018) Depression Symptoms and Warning Signs. Helpguide.org. January, 2018. https://www.helpguide.org/articles/depression/depression-symptoms-and-warning-signs.htm

[20] **Newberry A, et. al.** (2013) Exploring Spirituality in Family Caregivers of Patients With Primary Malignant Brain Tumors Across the Disease Trajectory Oncol Nurs Forum. 2013 May 1; 40(3): 10.1188/13.ONF.E119-E125. doi: 10.1188/13.ONF.E119-E125 https://www.ncbi.nlm.nih.gov/pmc/articles/PMC3880559/

[21] **Continuimn Health Partners, Inc**. Spiritual Needs. Net of Care Information and Resources for Caregivers. BethIsrael University Hospital and Manhattan Campus for the Albert Einstein College of Medicine. (copyrighted 2003-2005) http://www.netofcare.org/content/your_needs/spiritual_needs.asp

[22] **Alzheimer's Society.** (2015) Exercise Fact Sheet. (Downloadable PDF). http://www.alzheimers.org.uk/site/scripts/download_info.php?downloadID=1151

[23] **Cooke L.** (2015) Common Caregiving Mistakes. Lewy Warriors blog, Dec 2, 2015. https://lewywarriors.wordpress.com/category/life-as-a-caregiver/

[24] **Family Caregiver Alliance.** A Population at Risk. (2006) Family Caregiver Alliance, with California's Caregiver Resource Center.

[25] **Eldercare Locator.** (2018) Transportation Options for Older Adults and People with Disabilities. National Aging and Disability Transportation Center. Posted Jan 22, 2018. http://www.nadtc.org/resources-publications/transportation-options-for-older-adults-and-people-with-disabilities/

[26] **National Caregivers Library.** http://www.caregiverslibrary.org/

[27] **Bell, V and Troxel D.** (2013) The Best Friends Dementia Bill of Rights, 2013, Health Professionals Press, Inc. http://bestfriendsapproach.com/about/the-best-friends-bill-of-rights/

[28] **Crisis Prevention Institute.** (2016) Life Story Questionnaire. https://www.crisisprevention.com/CPI/media/Media/Specialties/dcs/Life-Story-Questionnaire.pdf

[29] **Macaulay S.** (2015) Teepa Snow demos 10 ways to de-escalate a crisis. August 28, My Alzheimer's Story. http://myalzheimersstory.com/2015/08/28/teepa-snow-demos-10-ways-to-calm-a-crisis-with-a-person-living-with-alzheimers-dementia/

[30] **Gitlin L, et. al.** (2012) Managing Behavioral Symptoms in Dementia Using Nonpharmacologic Approaches: An Overview. JAMA. 2012 Nov 21; 308(19): 2020–2029. doi: 10.1001/jama.2012.36918. http://www.ncbi.nlm.nih.gov/pmc/articles/PMC3711645/

[31] **National Collaborating Centre for Mental Health (UK).** (2007) Therapeutic Interventions For People With Dementia – Cognitive Symptoms And Maintenance Of Functioning. Dementia: NICE-SCIE Guideline on Supporting People With Dementia and Their Carers in Health and Social Care, #42-7. Leicester (UK): British Psychological Society; 2007. https://www.ncbi.nlm.nih.gov/books/NBK55462/

[32] **Gardner M.** (2016) The value of an occupational therapist for people with dementia. Dementia Alliance International. September 27, 2016 Blog. https://www.dementiaallianceinternational.org/occupational-therapists-and-dementia/

[33] **LSTV Big and Loud.** Lee Silverman Voice Treatment. LSVT Global. https://www.lsvtglobal.com/

[34] **Snyder P.** Treasures in the Darkness. Early LBD experiences. Review and buy here: http://astore.amazon.com/rollercoaster15-20?_encoding=UTF8&node=4

[35] **Memory People Facebook Page.** A closed group for dementia victims, their caregivers and advocates.

[36] **Schneider C.** (2006) Don't Bury Me...It Ain't Over Yet. Author House. http://www.lbdtools.com/shop_books.html

[37] **Oakley K.** (2009) Canadian Psychological Assn. Psychology Works Fact Sheet: Environmental Adaptations to Dementia. Canadian Psychological Assn. http://www.cpa.ca/docs/File/Publications/FactSheets/PsychologyWorksFactSheet_EnvironmentalAdaptationsToDementia.pdf

[38] **Bowes, A. et. al.** (2013) Physical activity for people with dementia: a scoping study. BMC GeriatricsBMC series ¿ open, inclusive and trusted201313:129. http://bmcgeriatr.biomedcentral.com/articles/10.1186/1471-2318-13-129 DOI: 10.1186/1471-2318-13-129

[39] **Wegerer J.** (2014) Nutrition and Dementia: Foods That May Induce Memory Loss & Increase Alzheimer's, Alzheimers.net 1/2/2014. http://www.alzheimers.net/2014-01-02/foods-that-induce-memory-loss/

[40] **Rettner R.** (2017) Meditation Really Does Lower Body's Stress Signals. Live Science, January 24, 2017. https://www.livescience.com/57618-meditation-lowers-stress-body.html

[41] **Bowen A.** (2014) Meditation for Caregivers. What, Why, and How to Get Started. Senior Advisor Blog, 11/2014. https://www.senioradvisor.com/blog/2014/11/meditation-for-caregivers-what-why-and-how-to-get-started/

[42] **Mozes A.** (2014) Yoga, Meditation May Help Dementia Patients. HealthDay News, June 5, 2014. WebMD News Archive. https://www.webmd.com/alzheimers/news/20140605/yoga-meditation-may-help-dementia-patients-and-caregivers-alike#1

[43] **Inner Health Studio.** Progressive Muscle Relaxation Audio and Active Physical Relaxation Techniques. Inner Health Studio, coping skills and relaxation resources. http://www.innerhealthstudio.com/muscle-relaxation-audio.html

[44] **Sauer A.** (2015) Manage Dementia's Side Effects with These 7 Essential Oils. Our Blog, August 10, 2015. Alzheimers.net. http://www.alzheimers.net/10-10-14-essential-oils-dementia/

[45] **ASPCA.** (2018) Is the Latest Home Trend Harmful to Your Pets? What You Need to Know! The American Society for the Prevention of Cruelty to Animals. January 17, 2018. https://www.aspca.org/news/latest-home-trend-harmful-your-pets-what-you-need-know

[46] **Christina.** (2015) The Science of Smell in Aromatherapy – How Smelling Essential Oils Works. The Hippy Homemaker. http://www.thehippyhomemaker.com/the-science-of-smell-in-aromatherapy-how-smelling-essential-oils-works/

[47] **Viggo H N**, et al. (2006) Massage and touch for dementia. Cochrane Database Syst Rev. 2006 Oct 18;(4):CD004989. http://www.ncbi.nlm.nih.gov/pubmed/17054228

[48] **British Acupuncture Council** (2013) Dementia. Back to Research Fact Sheet. March 28, 2013. http://www.acupuncture.org.uk/a-to-z-of-conditions/a-to-z-of-conditions/3202-dementia.html

[49] **Yang M-H**, et al. (2007) The efficacy of acupressure for decreasing agitated behavior in dementia: a pilot study. J Clin Nurs. 2007 Feb;16(2):308-15. http://www.ncbi.nlm.nih.gov/pubmed/17239066

[50] **Johnson J and Chow M.** (2015) Hearing and music in dementia. Handb Clin Neurol. 2015; 129: 667–687. doi: 10.1016/B978-0-444-62630-1.00037-8

[51] **Hamilton J.** (2014) Your Brain's Got Rhythm, And Syncs When You Think. All Things Considered, June 17, 2014. NPR. https://www.npr.org/sections/health-shots/2014/06/17/322915700/your-brains-got-rhythm-and-syncs-when-you-think

[52] **CTV News.ca.** (2016) The sound of healing: Study says sound-stimulation could help Alzheimer's patients. Health. CTV News. http://www.ctvnews.ca/health/the-sound-of-healing-study-says-sound-stimulation-could-help-alzheimer-s-patients-1.2868393

[53] **Bulsara C and Steuxner S.** (2012) Using Sound Therapy To Ease Agitation Amongst Persons With Dementia. The Brightwater Center. June 2012. https://www.fightdementia.org.au/sites/default/files/1530-Bulsara.pdf

[54] **Dark G.** (2016) Mandalas: A stress-busting art therapy. Daily Sabah Health. January 20, 2016. https://www.dailysabah.com/health/2016/01/21/mandalas-a-stressbusting-art-therapy

[55] **Aubrey A.** (2010) Mental Stimulation Postpones, Then Speeds Dementia. NPR News. September 4, 2010 http://www.npr.org/templates/story/story.php?storyId=129628082

[56] **Palmer L.** (ongoing) Picture books for those with dementia. A Listopia. https://www.goodreads.com/list/show/41392.picture_books_for_those_with_dementia

[57] **Jennings J.** (2012) Living with Lewy Body Dementia. One Caregiver's In-Depth Experience. 2012, WestBow Press. Blog: http://www.ourlewybodydementiaadventure.com/

[58] **Expert Blog.** (2012) Are pets a good idea for people with Alzheimer's? February 17, 2022. Home Instead Alzheimer's & Dementia Support. http://www.helpforalzheimersfamilies.com/2012/02/getting-a-pet/

[59] **Rossato-Bennett M.** (2014) Alive Inside. Documentary film. http://www.aliveinside.us

[60] **AmazingSusan.** (2016) 10 ways to use improv to improve life with alzheimer's.04/15/2016. My Alzheimer's Story. http://myalzheimersstory.com/2016/04/15/10-ways-to-use-improv-to-improve-life-with-alzheimers/

[61] **Schneider C.** (2006) Don't Bury Me...It Ain't Over Yet. Author House. (March 6, 2006). https://www.amazon.com/Dont-Bury-AINT-OVER-YET/dp/1425913954

Made in the USA
Coppell, TX
21 May 2021